# THE REAL FOOD SOLUTION

## ACHIEVE YOUR WEIGHT AND WELLNESS GOALS, INCREASE YOUR ENERGY AND GIVE YOUR FAMILY DELICIOUS REAL FOOD!

## WENDY McCALLUM

FORMAC PUBLISHING COMPANY LIMITED
HALIFAX

The information provided in this book is designed to provide helpful information on the subjects discussed. This information is not intended to be a substitute for professional medical advice, diagnosis or treatment. Always seek the advice of your physician or other qualified health provider with any questions about your medical condition. Do not disregard professional medical advice or delay seeking advice or treatment because of something you have read here.

Formac Publishing Company Limited recognizes the support of the Province of Nova Scotia through Film and Creative Industries Nova Scotia. We are pleased to work in partnership with the agency to develop and promote our creative industries for the benefit of all Nova Scotians. We acknowledge the support of the Canada Council for the Arts which last year invested $157 million to bring the arts to Canadians throughout the country.

 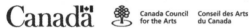 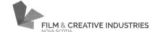

Cover design: Meghan Collins
Cover image: Jen Partridge

Library and Archives Canada Cataloguing in Publication

McCallum, Wendy, author
    The real food solution : achieve your weight and wellness goals, increase your energy and give your family delicious real food / Wendy McCallum.

Includes index.
Issued in print and electronic formats.
ISBN 978-1-4595-0394-6 (paperback).--ISBN 978-1-4595-0395-3 (epub)

    1. Cooking (Natural foods). 2. Cookbooks. I. Title.

TX741.M28 2016              641.5'637              C2015-904653-X
                                                   C2015-904654-8

Formac Publishing Company Limited
5502 Atlantic Street
Halifax, Nova Scotia, Canada
B3H 1G4
www.formac.ca

Printed and bound in Canada.

# Contents

## PART 4: TOOLS FOR SUCCESS

*Download more copies at
www.formaclorimerbooks.ca/realfood/mealplan.pdf.

# INTRODUCTION

Hello! I'm Wendy McCallum: real food coach and nutrition educator, cookbook author, happily recovering lawyer and the mom of two excellent, creative, active (and perpetually hungry) kids. Thanks for cracking open my latest book! I'll bet you're curious to see if there's anything different in here from all the other books you've read, and if this might finally be the approach that actually works for you. I'm also guessing you're a woman, most likely a fellow mom, and while you've got some changes you would like to make to your diet, you'd also love to improve your whole family's food. You've probably already started dabbling with "real" or "clean" food ingredients and recipes, but have yet to make very many changes that have stuck. You may even have tried some of the more popular extreme approaches to weight loss and wellness, such as paleo, gluten-free or vegan, but those changes were really hard to make and even harder to maintain, not to mention they might not have thrilled your whole family. Am I on the right track?

What you're really looking for is a simple, healthy approach that will work to get you to all your goals — whether we're talking about your personal weight and wellness or your family's food — and allow you to realistically maintain them for life. You want something that works with your family's busy life, while being flexible, kid-friendly and (gasp, dare you even wish it?) fun. You're not looking for a radical, instant solution, but instead have accepted the fact that real, lasting change, in the family kitchen and on the scale, comes with the slow and steady building of positive habits. If that sounds like you, I've got great news: this is *exactly* the book you are looking for.

# PART 1
# THE PLAN
# & PROGRAM

# CHAPTER 1

## What My Approach Can Do for You

What's different this time? Why will my program work for you when your other best efforts haven't led to lasting change? Because this time, you can actually do it, just like the hundreds of other real moms who have already used my approach to permanently lose weight, increase their energy and build better family food habits.

My program sets you up for success. It doesn't involve unpleasant deprivation, strange ingredients, weird flavours, superhuman kitchen skills or even fancy equipment. It's based on the time-tested truth that nothing too extreme or complicated ever works for very long. Let's face it: we're all leading really busy lives and need a straightforward, simple approach that will work for the whole family and keep us sane. No mom wants (or should have) to put more than one healthy meal on the table at a time. Who's got the time for that?

Most of the moms I meet and work with have two parallel food goals: to achieve and maintain a healthy weight and to get their whole family consistently eating better, less-processed food. Moms are frustrated by a diet industry that is often impractical and extreme, advocating a quick-fix approach. My program gives you everything you need to get yourself to a healthy body weight — or maintain it if you are already there — without eating different food from the rest of your family and without counting points, carbs or calories. If you're like most women of our generation, you grew up with a mother who was always on a diet. It's critical that we break that cycle for our children, and that's just another benefit of my approach: nobody even needs to know you're trying to lose weight. You'll sell the changes to your family for the really important reasons healthy food matters — increased energy, immunity and wellness. You'll role model healthy eating and use my tested, effective (and fun!) strategies to get your spouse and kids on board and involved. And you'll feel amazing about the benefits your whole family is enjoying.

When I say this program gives you everything you need, I mean *everything*, including:

- six weeks of flexible meal plans,
- grocery lists and shopping tips,
- loads of varied, simple scrumptious recipes,
- "healthy fast food" meal choices,
- effective ideas for picky eaters,
- strategies for talking to your kids about real food and getting them involved,
- school lunch solutions,
- time-saving kitchen tips,
- solutions for keeping it (mostly) real while travelling and
- the simple truths and guidelines you need for lifelong maintenance and balance.

You'll cook my delicious, simple and healthy real food family meals, and by quietly paying attention to your personal serving sizes and hunger cues, the extra weight will steadily melt away. Perhaps more importantly, as you're getting there you will see amazing side benefits: you'll feel your energy levels steadily rise until they become reliable and consistent on a daily basis, and you might just notice that you are getting sick less often and recovering faster from those colds and flus than you used to. You'll also develop a lifelong set of planning, cooking and eating habits that will set the basis for a permanently new "normal" at your family table — and that your children will take with them when they leave the nest. You'll embrace balance when it comes to food and shed any family-food-based "mom guilt" that you previously might have felt.

Sounds pretty great, doesn't it? It is, I promise you, and you can absolutely do this!

# CHAPTER 2

## *My Approach*

My approach is all about real food. It's a simple program designed to build a set of healthy, lifelong habits for you and your family. "Real" foods have one ingredient, or are made entirely of one-ingredient foods. If it doesn't need a label, or if it has a label with ingredients you can imagine growing in nature, chances are it's real. If it's got a label and a bunch of unpronounceable and unidentifiable ingredients, chances are it's not.

What could be simpler than a diet made up of real, pronounceable, readily available foods? And real food isn't just easy, it's also delicious. I've spent loads of time in the kitchen perfecting simple recipes with real ingredients that taste great so that you don't have to. You're about to become an expert at using a wide variety of real foods to make absolutely delicious and satisfying meals.

A real food diet will help you get to a healthy weight, but we all know permanent change comes only when we're motivated by more than the number on the scale. When I teach people about the real connection between food and energy levels, immunity and disease prevention, they start to notice the positive changes in their own wellness that come with improvements to their diet. This book will help you recognize these changes in your wellness — and you'll see them in family members too. You'll find it easier to maintain weight loss and continue your new habits, because you'll *feel* healthier. And who doesn't want that?

So what does this real food program really involve? Keeping it simple, I use the macronutrients (or "big nutrients") we need to stay alive as my food groups: carbohydrates, protein and fat. Once you're eating these three food groups in better balance, you'll experience increased energy, steady moods and more even blood-sugar patterns. This approach also keeps you feeling full for even longer and reduces carbohydrate and sugar cravings, which makes it so much easier to remain on track with healthy food choices. As an added bonus, it tends to keep the rest of your family on a more even keel. You'll even see more predictable behaviour from toddlers to teenagers!

Carbohydrates are our main source of fuel. Cars need gas; we need carbs. Good carbohydrates come in the form of veggies, fruits and whole grains, which provide a source of energy and fibre. They're also micronutrient-dense, meaning they're chock full of the "little nutrients" like vitamins, minerals, and phytonutrients that we need to stay healthy and energized. Most crackers, cookies, bagels, breads and processed snacks like pretzels give us carbs for energy, but they're full of refined sugars and white flour — usually low in fibre and relatively devoid of much other nutrition. For that reason, we're not counting these as real foods.

We need adequate protein to build and repair almost everything in our body. Protein is sort of like Lego: it comes in through our food in all different sizes, shapes and colours (the many amino acids), is then used immediately, or collected in a bin (your liver), grouped into task-specific blocks and sent out to wherever it's needed to build or rebuild. Kids' bodies are focused more on building (growing), but the older we get the more daily repair work our bodies need. If you're a typical Canadian family most of your protein is currently coming from meat and dairy, and you're probably eating a little too much of those animal foods. To balance this, I've suggested some tasty vegetarian protein alternatives you can easily incorporate into your weekly meals.

The often most neglected (yet oh-so important) macronutrient — healthy fat — is found in foods like nuts and seeds (and their butters), fish, flax and chia seeds, avocados and a variety of plant oils. Healthy fat gives your body what it needs to keep your cells healthy and help your immune system fight inflammation.

Since we're aiming for long-term change, the approach calls for balance — it's not an extreme or regimented diet. Most of the food your family eats will be real, but not *all* of it will be. Why not shoot for 100 per cent real food? As healthy and noble a goal as that might be, it's just plain impossible for most adults — let alone entire families — to maintain for very long. So don't aim for perfection: just 80 per cent or more of the real foods, with a 20 per cent or less allowance for the "not-so-perfect" foods built in. That means there's wiggle room for birthday cake, family celebrations, road trips, dining out, chocolate or your much-cherished Friday night glass of wine. The next couple of chapters will detail exactly how to achieve this balance for your family and why it will support increased energy, wellness and a healthy weight for life.

This is a plant-based program, but that doesn't mean you have to give up meat — just achieve a balance. People who eat more fruits and veggies feel better, are generally healthier and have a much easier time maintaining a healthy weight — and most of us just aren't eating enough. In my experience, the average Canadian family eats only three to five servings a day, while *really* healthy families eat seven to ten servings. In the chapters that follow, I'll show you how increasing your fruit and veggie intake fills up your "vitamin and mineral bank account," allowing you to create energy efficiently, support your immune system and decrease your risks of many of our most common chronic illnesses. I'll even give you the language you need to talk to your kids about why eating more plants really matters. This book is full of ideas for activities and challenges you can do with your kids to get them motivated and excited to make healthy changes and help with real food and cooking.

Because no two families are the same, this program is designed to be flexible. The right approach for you will be one that you enjoy and can easily keep up, and only you know what that is. If you're keen to start losing some weight right away, you can start following the program to the letter and ease your family in more gradually. Start with the popular and effective "Cleanstart" program, which I've included as one of the weekly meal plans in this book — following that for a week or two will really kickstart your weight loss and clean eating. Many moms find it's exactly what they need to get motivated and on track for healthy, permanent change. Others will want to start more gradually, keeping some foods (like gluten, sugar or dairy) in their diet in moderation by using the recipes and guidelines for balance in the meal plans.

In terms of your family's food, I recommend you start by trying some of the recipes and fun strategies I've provided in Chapter 10 for getting your kids (even the pickiest ones) excited and involved in your family's real food. The key to getting buy-in from your family is to give them a stake in your family food. Get them involved in meal planning, shopping, prep and cooking, set-up and cleanup, and praise them for their involvement and successes. Chapter 10 is filled with concrete ideas for getting kids of all ages involved, so use that as a resource to get you started.

Easing children (and even set-in-their-ways spouses) in with gradual change combined with education and positive reinforcement is the best way to steadily build a set of permanent healthier family habits. You can work towards your own weight and wellness goals without eating completely different food from everyone else, by serving everyone the same healthy main dish from the meal plan, but eating a little less and swapping the bread or pasta on their plates for more veggies or a salad on yours. To make this easy for you, I've included specific weight-loss portion sizes for all the recipes in the meal plans. This allows you to lose weight without any fuss, all the while role-modelling really great eating.

My recipes are all delicious and kid-friendly. They've been tested not only by my children but by hundreds of other families, and I regularly hear back from moms who are absolutely delighted with the feedback they're getting from their whole family on the food they're serving.

Working through my meal plans, you'll develop a repertoire of easy, healthy family favourites. You'll be able to start doing your own meal planning to incorporate those recipes into your life and schedule using the planning, organization and food prep tips provided in later chapters. You'll build up a freezer full of healthy "fast food" meals for those rushed evenings, taking the pressure off you and allowing you to enjoy more of that much-needed downtime at the table with your family.

The meal plans and recipes are also really easy to adjust to suit any specific dietary concerns or restrictions you might have in your family. While there are loads of gluten- and/or dairy-free meals, for example, you might choose to serve them to some or all of your family members topped with grated cheese or over pasta. If you like your morning coffee with milk and don't warm to the flavour of almond milk, choose cow's milk. If you've got a peanut allergy in your household, recipes that call for peanut butter can always be adapted by subbing in almond or sunflower seed butter. If you don't eat meat, choose from the many vegetarian options.

I've also built practical flexibility into the meal plans. For example, if you find yourself without the ingredients or time to make the meal on the plan for Monday, feel free to use a meal from any other day on the plan or something you have frozen from the week before. Just be sure to follow the recommended portion sizes if you're trying to lose weight. If only two of your family members were home to eat the chili last night, don't create unnecessary work for yourself — serve it up again tonight! If you're eating and cooking for one, freeze half of every recipe you make in single-serve portions and don't worry about eating the same lunch a couple of days in a row if that makes your life easier and reduces waste.

What do you have to lose? The extra weight, the low energy, the brain fog and the mom guilt you feel when you think about what your kids ate last week.

What will you gain? First, I'll reunite you with your kitchen and get you loving it again. After a few weeks of working at it, you'll notice the load start to lighten — not only will you be more familiar with the ingredients and recipes, you'll have a better-stocked pantry and meals frozen that you can incorporate into your weekly meal plans. You'll start losing weight, and your energy will climb back to that elusive pre-baby level. You'll feel fabulous about what you're doing for yourself and about what you're feeding your family.

Are you ready? Then let's get started!

# CHAPTER 3

# The 80/20 Rule: What It Is

The 80/20 Rule is my go-to approach to real food. When I start working with someone — whether they are young or old, sick or well, at a healthy weight or looking to lose — we begin by working towards 80/20. Its simplicity and basis in common sense make it appealing, but the bottom line is, it works. The built-in balance makes it an achievable goal, no matter how many you're cooking for.

Most families I work with are starting with a diet of about 50 per cent real, 50 per cent processed food. Some are doing a little better, some a little worse, but most have quite a few changes to make to get to 80 per cent real food. Start by gauging where you and your family are by tracking your food for a week and noting how much of what you are eating meets our criteria for real food. This will also give you a benchmark for change — tuck your food log away and pull it out in six months. You'll be impressed by your progress, and you'll see concrete evidence of how much your habits have changed for the better!

Let's take a closer look at some of the changes you'll be making. As I explained Chapter 2, the 80 per cent (or more) of real food is made up of three big food groups: healthy carbohydrates, protein and fat. Within each of those groups are hundreds of foods, so you'll have lots of variety to choose from. You're probably already eating a lot of these healthy, real foods — just not in the rights amounts. This program is designed to get you to exactly where you need to be for optimum balance.

Healthy, or "good," carbs are our preferred source of energy, and we could all use a little more of that! We get real, good quality carbs from three types of foods: veggies (my favourite), fruits and whole grains. We can also get carbohydrates (which is really just a fancy word for sugar) from other, less healthy sources, such as refined grain flours, sugary foods and alcohol. These foods might provide us with energy, but they don't give us much else.

When we take in carbohydrates in their healthy, real food form, they are wrapped in natural "goodness" in the form of fibre, vitamins and minerals. Now go back to my "Can you imagine it in nature?" test for a minute. You *can't* imagine white grains or flours in nature, because they don't grow that way. Picture wheat in a field: it's golden brown. Rice in nature is brown, black or red. To make these whole grains white, we need to remove the colour, which is the very place the "goodness" is usually found in natural food. We're left with naked carbs, stripped of their fibre, which provide us with little more than a quick boost of blood sugar followed by an equally fast plunge. Fruits and veggies of all kinds also package their carbs in goodness — colour — which is why they're a key part of a real food diet.

So, what healthy carbs will you be enjoying in abundance? *All* fruits and veggies, including a daily dose of leafy greens, flavour-packed fresh herbs, juicy berries and the occasional comforting sweet potato. You'll also enjoy whole grains like brown rice, quinoa and oats, as well as moderate amounts of whole grain flour products like whole wheat pitas, brown rice pasta and easy homemade tortillas. I've got some delicious salad dressing recipes lined up for you, and amazing soups and casseroles that will have you incorporating 7 to 10 servings of plants into your day without blinking.

What about real proteins? We need protein to build and repair cells, hormones and other essential parts on a daily basis. The majority of you get most of your daily protein from animal foods such as meat, fish, dairy and eggs. Unprocessed, one-ingredient versions of these foods fall into the 80 per cent category and are included in balance in the recipes and meal plans. Veggie protein options such as beans and legumes also fall into the 80 per cent category in their whole form. My goal is to get you eating animal foods in a healthier balance and incorporating lots of vegetable-based meals into your week. I'll also encourage you to look at where your animal-based foods are coming from, because what you picture when you "imagine them growing in nature" is often nothing like their actual living conditions. There are options available for more naturally raised meat, eggs and dairy; if you cut down on the amount you are eating you can afford better quality when you do buy them. And if you prefer to eat vegetarian or vegan, the program can easily be modified to suit your preferences.

The last 80 per cent real food category is healthy fat, which we need for all kinds of reasons, including cell and nerve health, and to combat inflammation. This is the category we hear about all too often in the media, and though it can seem confusing, it's really not all that complicated. Here's the skinny on healthy fat: artificial fats (like hydrogenated, partially hydrogenated and trans fats) are not healthy, and generally speaking, we need to eat more of the fat that comes from plants (as it is less present in our standard diet) than the fat that comes from animals. Of course, this is a generalization and there are exceptions, like the healthy fat we get from fish. Naturally raised animal fat in moderation is fine, but we need to work harder to include enough healthy plant-based fat. I've worked this in in small amounts in most of the meals and snacks on the plan: nuts and seeds, nut butters, healthy liquid plant oils like olive and flax oil, coconut oil, avocados and flax seeds will all become regulars in your rotation.

So what makes up the 20 per cent? Everything else. All the foods you eat that don't meet my guidelines for good carbs, protein and fat are the foods you'll be aiming to eat 20 per cent or less of the time.

Your family's 20 per cent will probably include things like sweets and sugary treats, processed convenient and fast foods, refined flour–based breads, pastas and crackers, white rice and alcohol.

Before you get too excited about eating 20 per cent junk, let's get real: when you're trying to lose weight, you'll be aiming for closer to a 95/5 ratio, because 80/20 probably won't get you all the way to your weight-loss goal. Following my 100 per cent real food meal plans and recipes, you'll reach your goal weight and use a moderated 80/20 (or better) approach once you're there to maintain your new, svelte self. The key is to find what fits best with your goals and lifestyle, which is why there's so much flexibility built into the program.

In the beginning, it might be challenging to limit these foods to 20 per cent or less, but as you get better at planning, shopping for and preparing delicious real food, it will get easier and easier. Your taste buds will slowly come down from the super-saturated sugar, salt and fat "high" they've been on and you'll start to really love, and even crave, the healthy stuff. After a few months of eating mostly real food, you'll indulge in your favourite restaurant dessert and it will taste so sweet just a few bites will be enough. Fast food and processed snacks will register as super-salty and not nearly as appealing. By the time you're a confirmed real foodie, your 20 per cent is going to look a lot different than it did when you started. Ten years ago I really loved a Cool Ranch Dorito (or thirty) and a big bowl of Cherry Garcia ice cream. Now I reach for a little dark chocolate with my glass of red, or some salsa and tortilla chips. My 20 per cent is more like 10 per cent, and there's not much artificial in there anymore.

The best part? I don't feel one bit deprived. And you won't either.

# CHAPTER 4

# The 80/20 Rule: Why It Works

If you haven't guessed by now, I'm a big fan of real food. Every day I see the amazing things it's doing for me, my family and the families I work with. It can take a couple of weeks of clean eating to see the benefits, so sometimes people need a little extra motivation in the beginning. So here it is — my simple, motivating explanation for why the 80/20 Rule boosts energy levels, strengthens immunity and overall wellness, and helps you maintain a healthy weight.

Picture a bright green piece of broccoli, where carbohydrate is surrounded by fibre and loads of micronutrients. Then consider a handful of jelly beans — what's wrapped around those sugary carbs? Usually a whole bunch of what I call non-food, like artificial colours, flavours and preservatives. Although that chemical cocktail is *technically* food (it's edible), it gives us absolutely nothing, nutritionally speaking — zero energy and no nutrients.

Your body doesn't much care where its main fuel source comes from. It's going to do pretty much the same thing with the sugars from the jelly beans as it does with the carbs in the broccoli: convert them to glucose and eventually into adenosine triphosphate, or ATP, which is our stored energy unit. It's also going to use pretty much the same metabolic processes in each case to do so. The key is that for that chain of metabolic events to occur, certain essential cofactors are required, most of which are B vitamins. Without them, your body can't convert sugar into useful energy, no matter how much you're eating.

Let's go back to the jelly beans. You pop them in your mouth, they move through your digestive tract and eventually their sugar is released into your blood. Your cells absorb the sugar and get busy trying to convert it into energy you can use. To do that, though, they need to have those essential B vitamins on hand, which they won't find in the jelly beans. So where do your cells get the B vitamins they need to metabolize the sugar in the candy? That's right — from the vitamins found in the real food in your diet, like broccoli.

Now, what does your body do with all the non-food in those jelly beans? It's got to get rid of it somehow, or else those artificial ingredients and toxins will need to be stored. So it starts a bunch of other processes in its detox systems to eliminate that garbage, and that all takes energy (more B vitamins) and often other vitamins and minerals as cofactors. Jelly beans don't give you any of these cofactors, so once again, your body's depending on real, nutrient-dense food like broccoli. I know I've used an extreme example of "not real" food with the jelly beans, but the truth is most processed food is devoid of or pretty low in nutrients (and if they're in there, they've often been artificially enriched).

Now let's consider the broccoli. When your body digests it, its sugar is also released into your blood, making its way to your cells, so they can convert it into energy. As you know, that process requires B vitamins, but guess what? In this real food example, they're right there, in the broccoli or the other real food you've eaten that day. It's easy to convert sugar to energy with the necessary cofactors packaged right alongside the carbs. And another bonus? Real food, like the broccoli, has no non-food ingredients that need to be dealt with.

Wondering what all this has to do with energy levels, wellness and healthy weight maintenance? Imagine a "vitamin and mineral bank account" in your body. (This is a very simplified analogy, but it really helps me get the point across, so bear with me. It's also an easy, effective way to explain why healthy eating matters to your kids.) When you're eating a pretty typical North American diet, consisting of 50 per cent processed and only 50 per cent real food, that bank account is probably running a bit low most of the time. It's not a severe deficit, but it's enough of one that when your cells are attempting to convert the abundance of sugar in your diet into useful energy, they find themselves searching for B vitamins to do so. The result is an inefficient and sluggish energy-creation process. Combined with the high-sugar and irregular eating patterns often present in a highly processed diet, as I explain in the next chapter, frankly it's no wonder you're feeling tired a lot of the time.

Of course, your immune system is also making regular "withdrawals" from your bank account, because it's highly reliant on vitamins and antioxidants. When your account's in the red, your immunity can suffer. You're far more likely to catch that nasty bug going around and a lot less likely to recover in time for the weekend.

When you get the balance right and you're eating at least 80 per cent real food and only 20 per cent or less of the not-so-great stuff, you're making regular daily deposits into your account. Your body always has what it needs to create energy and support a fully charged immune response, along with all the other essential functions it performs daily. This in turn supports a decreased risk of many of the most common chronic illnesses we face in North America today. That's how 80/20 improves energy and wellness.

What about maintaining a healthy weight? Most of those 80 per cent foods are lower in calories, sugar, sodium and unhealthy fat than the processed stuff. They're higher in fibre and far more nutrient-dense, which makes them more filling and satisfying. When you're eating 80 per cent of your diet from lower-calorie, filling foods, of course that naturally supports the maintenance of a healthy weight.

Feeling motivated? Let's start filling up your bank account!

# CHAPTER 5

## How to Eat

Real food, most of the time, really is the key. While that simple truth underpins my food philosophy, there are a few other important pieces of the puzzle that can really boost your chances of lifelong success. Obviously, you need to eat the right amount of real food — not too much and not too little — but you also need to eat it often enough, and in the right way, or eventually your blood sugar can get out of whack. When you have erratic blood-sugar patterns, your energy levels and mood suffer, and it can be harder to stay on track with your healthy, real food diet.

Here's the lowdown on blood sugar: carbohydrates digest faster than protein and fat. As you digest carb-based foods, especially the refined and processed ones, they dump their sugar into your blood in a hurry, causing your blood-sugar levels to spike. Your pancreas (or "blood-sugar watchdog") senses this and panics, because that kind of surge isn't supposed to happen. It reacts by pumping insulin into your blood. Imagine that each cell in your body has a door. Insulin is the key to the lock — without it, sugar can't enter your cells. When insulin floods into your blood following a sugar spike, all those doors are opened. This allows the sugar to move quickly into your cells, causing a rapid drop in your blood-sugar levels. Some of the sugar from your meal can be stored as glycogen in your liver and muscles, but the excess gets stored as fat in your cells. When your blood sugar drops, your pancreas releases another hormone, glucagon, which signals your liver to release stored glucose to bring your blood sugar back up. But when everything is working the way it should, your blood-sugar levels are properly regulated.

However, if you're suffering from hypoglycemia — low blood pressure — you can feel *awful*. Your brain feeds primarily off the glucose in your blood; when there's little there to absorb, your brain is hungry and doesn't function as well. Even when your blood-sugar regulation is working, you might get a headache, suffer from "brain fog" or feel sleepy, cranky or light-headed if you leave too long before eating, especially if your last meal was a really sugary or high-carb treat.

And while those symptoms are unpleasant, it's this that really does you in: you're so damn hungry you'd hand over your first-born for a chocolate chip muffin. Why are you craving starchy, sugary carbs? Because you know, from years of dedicated practise, that the fastest way to feel better is to eat more refined carbohydrates! Of course, if you do that, the nasty cycle just repeats and you soon feel rotten again. But if you possess superhuman willpower and resist that muffin without eating something healthy, you just get hungrier and hungrier. Eventually, it gets the best of all of us, and we cave and make a less-than-awesome food choice.

The key to staying on track with your food choices is to even out your blood-sugar curve by preventing those extreme highs and lows. Eliminating sugar spikes will also likely give you a more predictable, steady stream of energy as well as a more consistent mood — both of which are amazing bonuses. It will also reduce the likelihood of your cells becoming insulin-resistant in the future (with overuse, the lock can get sticky and insulin no longer opens cell doors effectively), which can lead to chronically elevated blood sugar and insulin and, eventually, type 2 diabetes. Yikes!

The good news is that supporting healthy blood-sugar patterns is easier than you think. The first step is to commit to a plant-based, real food diet, because fibre slows digestion and helps regulate the release of sugar into your blood. Plants, in the form of high-fibre veggies (along with moderate amounts of fruits and whole grains), will not only help you fill up your vitamin and mineral bank account, but will also deliver your energy more slowly and steadily. For those important reasons, you're going to work towards 7 to 10 servings of plants a day. This is built in to the meal plans, but if you're doing your own planning, incorporate this little trick: make it a non-negotiable rule that every time you eat, you'll include a veggie or a fruit. Assuming you are eating three meals and two snacks a day, that's a minimum of five plant servings daily. Next, get into the habit of serving at least two veggies with every family dinner. That takes you to six servings daily. With my recipes and meal ideas that squeeze veggies into surprising places, you'll find you can easily add another couple of servings.

Once you've started reducing blood-sugar spikes by choosing healthy, high-fibre carbs over sugary processed foods more often, it's time to really support your energy levels by getting into a couple more healthy habits. First, eat regularly — adopt a zero-tolerance meal-skipping policy. Next, avoid eating carbs (even the good ones) alone.

Let's start with regular meals and snacks, and why this habit matters. If you're a meal skipper, stop now. The longer you leave between eating, the more likely you are to get hungry. That's not rocket science, right? The best policy is to eat three meals a day and have a couple of small, balanced snacks when you need them most. Snack time is flexible. Some people don't need a morning snack, but start to crash mid-afternoon. Others can't make it through the evening without a little healthy nosh to get them to morning. Some need a pre- or post-workout snack. Some work shifts and eat their meals at different (albeit still regular) hours. Adopt whichever approach allows you to avoid getting to the point of that starving feeling. Your goal is to eat what you need to stay satisfied until just before the time of your next scheduled snack or meal. In other words, you should be getting hungry and be ready to eat when it's time to do so. Hunger cues are an important part of healthy, balanced eating, but a lot of us have lost them through years of meal skipping, overeating and dieting.

It's pretty much just common sense — if you're not hungry at a regular mealtime, you likely ate too much at your last sitting. If you're starving, you need to be eating more, or more regularly. The meal plans in this book promote regularly eating three meals and two snacks daily — more if you are very active, breastfeeding, a male or just find yourself getting too hungry too often. Pay attention to your personal hunger cues and adjust accordingly. When you find your balance, you can lose weight without losing your mind!

Next, get into the habit of avoiding carbs on their own, especially the really sugary, refined ones. When you eat a store-bought, "low-fat" chocolate chip muffin, you're taking in a lot of sugar, not much fibre and little to no protein or healthy fat. That muffin speeds through your system, causing the chain-reaction cycle of a blood-sugar spike, a panic reaction from your pancreas, followed by a drop in blood sugar, and a correction of blood-sugar levels by glucagon.

By choosing different foods, we can create a different picture. Let's say you have some scrambled eggs with sautéed veggies and sliced avocado for breakfast. You're eating carbs, but this time they're the good ones, with built-in fibre and nutrients, which moderately slow down digestion and the release of sugar. Both the egg and avocado contain protein and fat, and protein and fat take longer to digest than carbohydrate, keeping you satisfied longer. Instead of a reacting to a dump of sugar into your blood, your pancreas has time to react and manage the calm movement of sugar into your cells. It's a much less frantic response, which allows for a more moderate increase in blood sugar, a regulated cell uptake of sugar and a gradual decrease in blood sugar.

The trick, then, is to pair your healthy carbs with some protein and good fat whenever you can. Of course, I'm not leaving you to figure this out all on your own — my recipes and meal and snack combinations do this for you. Eventually, after some practise and time to familiarize yourself with easy ways to accomplish this, you'll start doing this pairing on your own. For example, instead of an apple alone (carb), have some natural peanut butter on it (protein and healthy fat); instead of baby carrots on their own (carb), pair them with some hummus for a hit of protein and healthy fat. A bowl of white rice and steamed veggies is a high-carb, lower-protein meal. Switch to whole grain brown rice, stir-fry those veggies in coconut oil and add some protein like chicken, shrimp or organic tofu, and now you've got a balanced meal that will keep you going a lot longer.

So, here's the key to real food satisfaction: we need to prevent sugar spikes and willpower-sapping hunger by eating real food regularly, choosing healthy carbs, and eating protein and healthy fat with those carbs whenever we can. That means steadier energy levels, increased meal satisfaction, more predictable moods and decreased cravings, all of which support steady weight loss and maintenance. Combined with my delicious, real food recipes, this way of eating is something you can truly enjoy and embrace for life.

So now you're armed with all the information you need — jump in and get started!

# CHAPTER 6

## The Program

### GETTING STARTED

Now that you've got the fundamentals of why you're making a change to a real food diet, let's talk about how to get started. The key to lasting success is to get really good at preparing and organizing your real food. For most of you, this will mean developing new systems and habits when planning meals, grocery shopping and cooking. The important steps you need to take are set out in this chapter and the next, so read them both carefully.

Following these steps, you'll become efficient in all areas of real food prep (both in and out of the kitchen). It might seem at first like you're spending more time planning, shopping and cooking, but as your habits change this will all become easier, and these changes have a huge payoff. You'll not only start reaping the rewards of a diet rich in veggies and fruits and supportive of balanced blood sugar, but you'll also be a lot less stressed about what both you and your family are eating, and you'll feel organized, energized and motivated.

Before you get started, make a commitment to yourself to really prioritize healthy eating and lifestyle changes. I always say that the healthiest people are just a little bit selfish. Of course (especially for us moms), this does not come easily. But if you don't put your health and wellness first, who will? This is a really important step in becoming healthier and happier. Take some time to write down your goals — and try to make most of them unrelated to the scale. Of course, it's important to establish a realistic, healthy weight that you would like to achieve and maintain, but you need more than a number on a scale to motivate you to make lasting, positive change.

What other benefits are you hoping to gain? Are you hoping your skin will improve as a result of a cleaner diet? Maybe you'd like to improve the quality and duration of your sleep, or are looking forward to big improvements in your energy levels. If you and your family members are constantly getting sick, isn't strengthening everyone's immunity something awesome to look forward to? How about the importance of raising healthy eaters, who leave for college armed with the knowledge, habits and skills to continue eating well for life? Maybe you just want to have the energy to play with your kids outside, or teach them how to ski, or just get yourself to that yoga class more often. There are *so* many great reasons to eat well for life. I really encourage you to identify all of the other amazing benefits you'd love to see before you get started on this program. Write them down, and revisit that list often. It will keep you motivated and on track on the days the scale doesn't.

Obviously, with your whole family on board, spending the time you need to ensure you're eating great food no longer seems selfish, because everyone benefits. It's really important to start talking to your partner and children about the exciting, healthy changes you're going to be undertaking together. For tips and tricks for getting buy-in from your family, spend some time going through Chapter 10 — I've even included kid-friendly language to use and fun ways to get everybody involved in your family's food.

Once you've made this commitment and talked with your family, the next step is to set yourself up for success, which includes getting your pantry and kitchen stocked, and your meal plan and grocery list for the week ready.

Before you do any planning or shopping, get your kitchen and pantry cleaned out and organized. Set aside an afternoon or evening to clean out your fridge, freezer and pantry, getting rid of all of the expired foods and any processed, unhealthy ingredients that will only tempt you. You don't need to get rid of all the treats in your house — there's a place for those in every balanced diet — but if you have a weakness for junk food, make the transition easier for yourself by removing the temptation. Another good idea is to go through your Tupperware drawer and sort out the containers that no longer have lids or are looking a little worse for wear. I like to store and freeze food in ovenproof glass containers, Mason jars and BPA-free plastic containers or zip-top bags. If, after cleaning out your drawer, it looks like you're in short supply of these freezer-friendly items, it's time to restock so you're in good shape to start prepping, cooking and freezing, as well as packing your lunches and snacks if you work out of the home during the day.

After you've cleaned, it's time to restock. I've provided *everything* you need to get prepared in Chapter 9, so go through those supports and tools carefully before you get started. Review the detailed Pantry, Fridge and Freezer Staples List (pages 170–180), which sets out all of the basic condiments and ingredients you'll use on a regular basis in my recipes. You probably already have a lot of these foods on hand, but stock up on any you don't before starting the program. You'll need to spend some extra money at the grocery store in the first month or so as you build up your staple ingredients, but once you have a well-stocked pantry, you'll find your grocery bills rebalance. If you want to follow a meal plan to the letter, I recommend that you have most of the items on the Staples List before you start. (These basic ingredients are generally not included in the weekly grocery list that goes with each plan.) If you're easing yourself into more real food by incorporating a few of my recipes into your week, you can just go through those recipes carefully and purchase what you need as you need it.

Review the list of kitchen tools in Chapter 9, and identify what you might benefit from adding to your own kitchen. Most of the tools are relatively inexpensive, and are well worth your money in terms of the time they will save you in food prep. The bigger ticket items, like a good quality food processor, can often be found on sale and also make great gifts on birthdays, Mother's Day and Christmas, so add them to your list!

Once you've stocked up on staples and kitchen supplies, it's time to start meal planning, using all of the tips and tools I've provided in Chapter 9. You'll even find information on how to plan, where to shop (on a budget) and how to save time prepping and cooking so that you can enjoy the rest of your life.

Because this program is flexible, you have several options for getting started. If you want to kickstart weight loss and increase energy levels, start with a week or more of my Cleanstart Program (page 42). Read the detailed introduction (Welcome to Cleanstart! — immediately following this section) to that week of meal planning to determine if it's right for you. If not, choose a different week of meal planning that appeals to you, and get organized using all the tools I've provided to follow it. The other meal plans are less restrictive than the Cleanstart week, so they may provide a more realistic happy medium for you. If you're brand new to the concept of real food, or just prefer to go one step at a time, start by choosing a couple of recipes that appeal and simply incorporate those into your regular family meals. You can gradually increase your repertoire of healthy food, and decrease the processed food in your family's diet in the process.

There is also flexibility built right into each weekly meal plan, which provides for breakfast, lunch, dinner and two snacks daily. Breakfasts are always interchangeable with any other breakfast in the week (or even in any other weekly meal plan), and the same goes for lunches and dinners. This allows you to choose the recipes and meals you feel like eating, and also to effectively use up any leftovers or premade, frozen meals that you might have stocked in your freezer. You will also have a list of healthy snacks to choose from, and can choose two (or more, if necessary) of the snacks on a daily basis. You'll probably find you naturally gravitate towards some of the snack choices more often than others, and that's fine. If there's a night where you just can't get it together to make what you'd planned, don't panic. Choose from one of the "healthy fast food" meals on page 169 and give yourself a break!

The weekly meal plans can easily be tailored to individuals with special dietary needs, including the need for increased calories. If you're breastfeeding, extremely active or a male, for example, you'll simply need to eat more of the real foods set out in the meal plan. Start by increasing your portion sizes by about 25 per cent, and then pay attention to hunger cues to see whether this is enough, or possibly too much, of an increase. You should be hungry and ready for your next meal, but absolutely never starving, or feeling any of the symptoms we would associate with that, such as lightheadedness or a headache.

If you're a vegetarian, and the weekly meal plan includes recipes with meat, simply substitute any other vegetarian recipe from the program's recipe collection. There are many delicious vegetarian options to choose from, all clearly identified so you can find them easily.

Whatever option you choose, you'll take the same basic steps to make sure you're organized and set up for success. First, as I suggested above, you need to go through the Staples List and make sure your pantry is stocked. I assume each week that you have maintained a stocked pantry and are replacing the basic ingredients on the Staples List when your supply starts to run low.

Next, go through the grocery list that accompanies your meal plan, or if you're just incorporating a few specific recipes, go through those recipes carefully and make sure that you have added whatever items you need to your weekly grocery list. Depending on how many family members will be following the meal plan, you will need to increase the amounts of certain foods from the grocery lists, for example, protein (such as chicken, fish and tofu amounts), produce and snack items.

You'll see that each weekly meal plan is set up with the assumption that most of you have more flexibility with your time on the weekends and will prefer to do your big weekly grocery shop and prep on Saturday and/or Sunday. However, if you tend to work weekends or shiftwork, this may not be the case for you. If you're retired, you probably prefer to do your grocery shopping during the week, when the stores are less busy. Day 1 might be a Monday or any other day. The key is to make sure that whenever your Day 1 is, you have had adequate time to prepare for it in the days prior by meal planning, grocery shopping and doing the suggested prep.

After you've been to the grocery store, take a look at the suggestions for advance prep at the beginning of the meal plan you're following, and set a little time aside to make sure you get that completed. This will ensure that you're starting the week off on the right foot, that your first day is not overwhelming and that you get up and do it again the next day! You'll see that I often suggest some prep in the evenings or on the weekends to make the next day go smoother — it's generally worth it to spend a few minutes in the evening getting ready for the next day, and this will eventually become a habit that will serve you well for life!

## WELCOME TO CLEANSTART!

Why is Cleanstart a great first week meal plan? Because committing to a week (or two) of 100 per cent real food is great way to kickstart a healthy-eating or weight-loss program, or to get yourself back on track after a period of excess or less-than-healthy eating. After a few days on Cleanstart, you'll feel start to feel lighter, less bloated and more energetic and focused than you have for a long time. As an added bonus, most followers lose three to five pounds by the end of the first week!

This week is stricter than the rest of the program's meal plans. It is a completely dairy-, sugar- and gluten-free *really* clean week of eating that's designed to give your body a break from high-sugar, processed and other commonly irritating foods. You will begin to restore a balance in your digestive tract between good and bad bacteria, which may be upset by years of poor diet, antibiotic use and many other factors.

Of course, if you've been eating the standard North American diet for years, rebalancing your gut takes a lot longer than a week. That's what the rest of the program (and the rest of your real food life) is for!

While the Cleanstart meal plan is only one week long, you may decide to stay with it for another week or two once you start to experience its benefits. It's totally up to you, but I don't believe it's a great idea for anyone to try to follow it for too long because it's relatively restrictive. Instead, I recommend you move to one of the more moderate meal plans as soon as you start to feel like you're missing the restricted foods enough that you are no longer enjoying your food.

Cleanstart is a lot easier to stick to if you are prepared. I have included a grocery list for this week, as I have for all other weeks, and would suggest that you stock your fridge, freezer and pantry with those foods before you get started. As always, I assume you've gone through the Staples List (pages 170–180) and made sure you are well stocked with those foods. (You'll need most staples on that list, with the exception of gluten-containing foods, dairy, maple syrup, honey, vinegars other than apple cider vinegar, natural peanut butter and a few others that are restricted this week.) The Cleanstart-week grocery list includes the ingredients you'll need *aside from* those on the Staples List.

Many people, especially first-timers, experience a few days of mild effects as their bodies start reaping the benefits of being nourished with only real food on the Cleanstart week. Symptoms may include mild headaches, lethargy and aching or irritability, along with increased bowel activity. These symptoms are normal and let you know that your body is responding. They normally subside after the first few days. Your best bet to get through this is to drink lots of water, move your body with moderate exercise and get a good night's sleep.

• So, what's the deal with Cleanstart? If you can't eat gluten, dairy or sugar, what can you eat? Lots! Here's a list of the foods you'll be eating: You can eat all the veggies you want, so go nuts! Visit your local market or produce section and buy whatever strikes your fancy, with a focus on dark green and colourful vegetables. The goal should be to eat mostly vegetables this week, which may be a very new concept to you. Potatoes, sweet potatoes, corn and popcorn are also allowed, and avocadoes are permitted in moderation. I recommend you stick to a maximum of one serving of starchy veggies a day, and remember that avocado, while rich in healthy fat, is also high in calories.

- Non-gluten whole grains are permitted, with a special focus on brown rice. Other great grains to incorporate include oats, quinoa, millet and buckwheat. Eat these in their whole form — that is, avoid all flours and pastas. You can have some white rice, but should choose brown whenever you can. You can also occasionally eat brown rice cakes as a bread replacement with soup or salad this week.

- You can enjoy moderate amounts of good quality lean meat, fish, shellfish and eggs. Favour fish this week, but a little beef, chicken or pork is fine (just not in a processed form such as deli meat, sausage or bacon). Avoid farmed salmon (choose wild instead); it's full of all the stuff you are trying to get rid of!

- Legumes are great — again, in moderation — so you can include chickpeas (an ingredient in hummus), lentils, kidney and white beans, et cetera in your diet. You can also eat plain tofu (I always recommend buying organic to avoid genetically modified soybeans).

- You can have unsweetened almond, rice, soy or coconut milk (check your labels), but no cow's dairy products except for a little natural butter.

- You can also eat nuts and seeds (but not peanuts, as they often contain naturally occurring yeast and moulds, which are better avoided this week), with a focus on the non-oily nuts like almonds. Since tahini, one of the main ingredients in hummus, is made of sesame seeds, you can have hummus. Prepare it yourself using the Easy Hummus recipe (page 145). Natural, unsweetened almond butter (similar to peanut butter) is fine, but peanut butter needs to be avoided.

- You can enjoy one or two low-sugar fruits a day. These include apples, pears, strawberries, blueberries, raspberries, blackberries, peaches, apricots, nectarines and plums.

- Tea and coffee are also permitted (I hear your sigh of relief). Just stick to one to two cups in the morning, avoid artificially sweetened or flavoured versions, and don't add dairy (try unsweetened almond milk instead) or sugar (stevia in moderation is permitted).

- Try nutritional or vegetarian yeast. Don't know what this is? It's a flaky, yellow, cheesy-tasting ingredient you'll find in the natural foods section of the grocery story. It's safe on the cleanse and adds great flavour, protein and vitamin B12 to sauces and stir-fries, and is also great on popcorn.

- You can use all oils except peanut oil. Coconut oil is great for cooking at a high temperature, olive oil is perfect for lower than medium-heat cooking and flax is great for cold salad dressings (with lemon juice or apple cider vinegar).

- Herbs and spices are all acceptable and really are essential to enjoying the foods on this plan. Garlic, onions and other veggies from that family are all highly recommended, as they have great immune-supporting benefits and are packed with flavour. Include them whenever you can.

- Apple cider vinegar is the only permitted vinegar during Cleanstart. Look for one that specifically indicates is "with mother" on the label to get all the positive health benefits.

- Lemons/limes and lemon/lime juice are acceptable. Use grated rind and juice to flavour veggies and soups, and the juice with oil for salad dressing.

- Lacto-fermented veggies are allowed. Huh? No idea what these are? They include foods such as sauerkraut and kim chi (pickled cabbage), and help restore healthy gut bacteria. If you want to give these a go, look for them at your local health food store.

- Popcorn is permitted as long as it's stove-popped or air-popped, and makes a delicious snack. I recommend popping it on the stove in coconut oil.

If it's not on this list, chances are it's not Cleanstart-friendly, so I recommend you avoid it. You may choose to follow the Cleanstart seven-day meal plan I've provided to the letter, use it as a general guide or do your own thing altogether and design a unique meal plan within the guidelines. There are loads of "Cleanstart-friendly" recipes other than those listed in the meal plan. They're included in the recipes section, and clearly labelled "CF," so you've got lots of variety to choose from!

When you're ready to move to a more moderate form of clean eating, I recommend you reintroduce gluten and dairy one at a time, giving yourself a chance to notice any response your body might have to each food in isolation. If one reintroduced food doesn't bother you after a few days, introduce another. That will allow you to identify any sensitivities you might have, and you can then eliminate or reduce that food in your diet. For example, many people find that when they reintroduce dairy they immediately have uncomfortable symptoms of bloating or gassiness. I take a common sense approach to food sensitivities: if it bothers you, don't eat it! Whatever nutritional benefits a food might have, they can almost always be found in a just-as-healthy, non-irritating substitute.

# PART 2
# THE MEAL PLANS

# CHAPTER 7

# Cleanstart Week Meal Plan

## Before you start the week, make:

- Easy Hummus, p. 145
- Brown Rice (make a large batch from 3 cups dry rice, refrigerate half and freeze the remainder in 1/2 cup portions)
- Green Goddess Dressing, p. 143
- Beta Butternut Soup, p. 100
- Simple Chili, p. 119 (optional make-ahead, for Day 1 dinner)
- Hard boil 6 or more eggs
- Consider cleaning and chopping some of your greens and veggies in advance for snacks and salads during the week

## Preparing for the week

I encourage you to go through the meal plan and recipes carefully, using this list and the Staples List as tools to determine what you already have and what you still need to make this week a success. If you are cooking for more than one, you will need to increase amounts for accompaniments like salads and rice as well as snacks. The lunch and dinner recipes generally serve a family, but where a separate protein is called for (such as chicken, fish and/or tofu), you will also need to scale amounts for your group.

## Grocery list of additional items

Please refer to the pantry, fridge and freezer staples list (pages 170–180 for weekly basics

○ 1 large container prewashed spinach
○ 1 large container salad greens (any type)
○ 1 bunch kale, collards or chard
○ 2 butternut squash
○ 5 sweet potatoes or yams
○ 2 white potatoes
○ 5 yellow onions
○ 1 red onion
○ 1 bunch green onions
○ 1 ginger root (Buy one root, peel entire root before using and store remainder well wrapped in freezer for next time.)
○ 1 bunch asparagus
○ 1 large (or 2 small) head broccoli
○ 2 to 3 garlic bulbs
○ 1 large bag carrots (2 lb)
○ 1 head celery
○ 3 limes
○ 4 lemons
○ 1 avocado
○ 2 cucumbers
○ 2 medium tomatoes
○ 1 package grape tomatoes
○ 4 to 6 medium beets
○ 2 cups brussels sprouts
○ 1 napa cabbage
○ 1 green cabbage
○ 1 small purple cabbage
○ extra veggies for snacks, topping salads and rounding out stir-fries, as needed
○ 5 to 7 apples
○ 5 to 7 pears
○ 1 large bag frozen (or 2 containers fresh) berries
○ 1 bunch fresh parsley (any type)
○ 1 bunch fresh cilantro

○ 1 package fresh mint (you need 1/2 cup)
○ fresh rosemary (optional)
○ 1 can (28 oz/798 mL) crushed tomatoes
○ 2 cans (each 14 oz/398 mL) black beans
○ 1 can (14 oz/398 mL) kidney beans
○ 5 cans (each 14 oz/398 mL) chickpeas
○ 1 can (28 oz/798 mL) pumpkin purée (unsweetened)
○ 2 (each 900 mL) containers low-sodium vegetable stock
○ 3 to 4 boneless chicken breasts (optional, you may choose tofu instead)
○ 1 to 2 roasting chickens
○ white fish fillets (optional)
○ 2 to 3 blocks organic firm tofu (optional, you may choose chicken instead)
○ 2 dozen eggs
○ oat bran
○ natural almond butter (only ingredient should be almonds)
○ apple butter (no sugar added)
○ poultry seasoning (a spice)
○ stevia (powdered natural sweetener)
○ 2 cups raw almonds
○ 1/2 cup raw cashews
○ 1 cup popcorn kernels
○ 1 package brown rice cakes
○ 2 L unsweetened almond milk

| Day | Breakfast | Lunch | |
|-----|-----------|-------|---|
| 1 | **Cinnamon Oats & Berries**<br><br>1 serving Cinnamon Oats & Berries, p. 86<br><br>coffee or tea (with unsweetened dairy alternative such as almond or soy milk, and stevia, if you need sweetener) | **Beta Butternut Soup & Big Salad**<br><br>1 1/2 cups Beta Butternut Soup, p. 100<br><br>with a Big Salad: 2 cups salad greens, 1/2 cup chopped cooked chicken, tofu or beans of choice, 1 cup chopped raw veggies of choice, 1–2 tsp pumpkin or sunflower seeds or slivered almonds, 2 tbsp Green Goddess Dressing, p. 143 | |
| 2 | **Eggs with Sautéed Greens & Avocado**<br><br>1 serving Eggs with Sautéed Greens & Avocado, p. 87<br><br>1/2 cup berries<br><br>coffee or tea (with unsweetened dairy alternative such as almond or soy milk, and stevia, if you need sweetener) | **Simple Chili & Brown Rice Cake**<br><br>1 cup Simple Chili, p. 119<br><br>1 brown rice cake with 1 tbsp apple butter<br><br>1 apple or pear | |
| 3 | **Pumpkin Pie Baked Oatmeal**<br><br>1 serving warmed Pumpkin Pie Baked Oatmeal (p. 91) topped with 1/2 cup fresh or frozen berries and 1 tbsp chopped walnuts<br><br>Note: Make sure you sweeten this recipe with stevia during Cleanstart week!<br><br>coffee or tea (with unsweetened dairy alternative such as almond or soy milk, and stevia, if you need sweetener) | **Beta Butternut Soup & Big Salad**<br><br>1 1/2 cups Beta Butternut Soup, p. 100<br><br>with a Big Salad: 2 cups salad greens, 1/2 cup chopped cooked chicken, tofu or beans of choice, 1 cup chopped raw veggies of choice, 1–2 tsp pumpkin or sunflower seeds or slivered almonds, 2 tbsp Green Goddess Dressing, p. 143 | |

| Dinner | Snacks | Evening Prep |
|---|---|---|
| **Simple Chili over Brown Rice**<br><br>1 cup Simple Chili, p. 116<br><br>served over 1/2 cup brown rice<br><br>with raw veggies or side<br><br>salad: 1 cup greens, 1/2 to 1 cup chopped raw veggies of choice and 1 tbsp Green Goddess Dressing, p. 144<br><br>apple or 1/2 cup berries<br><br>*set aside 1 cup Simple Chili for tomorrow's lunch | Choose 2 Cleanstart snacks (or more, if you're really hungry) from the list at the end of this meal plan (p. 46). | Plan out 2 Cleanstart snacks a day, or more if you're really hungry — see list at the end of this meal plan (p. 46). |
| **Grilled Chicken, Fish or Tofu with Oven-Roasted Veggies & Side Salad**<br><br>4 oz chicken or fish or 1/4 of a 454 g block of organic tofu, brushed with a little olive oil and garlic then grilled or pan-cooked<br><br>1 cup Oven-Roasted Veggies, p. 115<br><br>with side salad: 1 cup greens, 1/2 to 1 cup chopped raw veggies of choice and 1 tbsp Green Goddess Dressing, p. 143 | Choose 2 Cleanstart snacks (or more, if you're really hungry) from the list at the end of this meal plan (p. 48). | Make Pumpkin Pie Baked Oatmeal (p. 91) for tomorrow morning's breakfast. |
| **Karmic Buddha Bowls**<br><br>1 serving Karmic Buddha Bowls, p. 122<br><br>*set aside 1 serving of Buddha Bowls for tomorrow's lunch | Choose 2 Cleanstart snacks (or more, if you're really hungry) from the list at the end of this meal plan (p. 48). | If tomorrow night is busy, premake Club Med Burgers (p. 120) and refrigerate, then reheat for tomorrow's dinner. |

| Day | Breakfast | Lunch | |
|---|---|---|---|
| 4 | **Take It To Go!**<br><br>2 hard-boiled eggs<br><br>1 cup berries or 1 apple or pear<br><br>coffee or tea (with unsweetened dairy alternative such as almond or soy milk,<br><br> and stevia, if you need sweetener) | **Karmic Buddha Bowls**<br><br>1 serving Karmic Buddha Bowls | |
| 5 | **Cinnamon Oats & Berries**<br><br>1 serving Cinnamon Oats & Berries, p. 86<br><br>coffee or tea (with unsweetened dairy alternative such as almond or soy milk, and stevia, if you need sweetener) | **Club Med Burger & Soup**<br><br>1 Club Med Burger, p. 120<br><br>1 tbsp Easy Hummus, p. 145, as garnish<br><br>1 cup Smoky Broccoli Soup, p. 99<br><br>*set aside a serving of Smoky Broccoli Soup for tomorrow's lunch | |
| 6 | **Southwestern Black Bean Frittata**<br><br>1 serving Southwestern Black Bean Frittata, p. 96<br><br>1 cup berries or 1 apple or pear<br><br>coffee or tea (with unsweetened dairy alternative such as almond or soy milk, and stevia, if you need sweetener) | **Smoky Broccoli Soup & Chickpea Tabbouleh**<br><br>1 cup Smoky Broccoli Soup, p. 99<br><br> 1 cup Chickpea Tabbouleh, p. 106 | |

| Dinner | Snacks | Evening Prep |
|---|---|---|
| **Club Med Burgers & Big Salad**<br><br>1 Club Med Burger, p. 120<br><br>1 tbsp Easy Hummus, p. 145, as garnish<br><br>with a Big Salad: 2 cups salad greens, 1/2 cup chopped cooked chicken, tofu or beans of choice, 1 cup chopped raw veggies of choice, 1–2 tsp pumpkin or sunflower seeds or slivered almonds, 2 tbsp Green Goddess Dressing, p. 143<br><br>1/2 cup berries or half an apple or pear | Choose 2 Cleanstart snacks (or more, if you're really hungry) from the list at the end of this meal plan (p. 48). | If tomorrow night is busy, peel and dice your squash for the Southwestern Black Bean Frittata (p. 96) and refrigerate and consider premaking Smoky Broccoli Soup (p. 99). |
| **Southwestern Black Bean Frittata & Grilled Veggies**<br><br>1 serving Southwestern Black Bean Frittata, p. 96<br><br>4 to 6 grilled asparagus spears (trim tips off asparagus, toss with 1 tsp olive oil and roast at at 375°F on baking sheet about 10 minutes or until tender).<br><br>1 apple or pear<br><br>*set aside a serving of Frittata for tomorrow's breakfast | Choose 2 Cleanstart snacks (or more, if you're really hungry) from the list at the end of this meal plan (p. 48). | If tomorrow is busy, make Chickpea Tabbouleh (p. 106) for tomorrow's lunch. |
| **Stir It Up!**<br><br>1 serving Stir It Up! with Nutty Lime or Simple Stir-fry Sauce, p. 139<br><br>Served over 1/2 cup brown rice or quinoa | Choose 2 Cleanstart snacks (or more, if you're really hungry) from the list at the end of this meal plan (p. 48). | |

| Day | Breakfast | Lunch | |
|-----|-----------|-------|---|
| 7 | **Pumpkin Pie Baked Oatmeal**<br><br>1 serving warmed Pumpkin Pie Baked Oatmeal (p. 91) topped with 1/2 cup fresh or frozen berries and 1 tbsp chopped walnuts<br><br>Note: Make sure you sweeten this recipe with stevia during Cleanstart week!<br><br>coffee or tea (with unsweetened dairy alternative such as almond or soy milk, and stevia, if you need sweetener) | **Smoky Broccoli Soup & Chickpea Tabbouleh**<br><br>1 cup Smoky Broccoli Soup, p. 99<br><br>1 cup Chickpea Tabbouleh, p. 106 | |

## Snacks: Cleanstart week

- 1/4 cup Easy Hummus (p. 145) with raw veggies
- 1 brown rice cake with 1 tsp each natural almond butter and apple butter
- 1 hard-boiled egg with 1 cup cherry tomatoes
- 1 sliced apple with 1 tsp natural almond butter or 12 almonds
- 1 cup berries with 1 cup unsweetened almond or soy milk
- 3 cups homemade popcorn (air-popped or popped in small amount of coconut oil)
- 1 brown rice cake with 1 tbsp Easy Hummus (p. 145) and 1/8 of an avocado, sliced

| Dinner | Snacks | Evening Prep |
|---|---|---|
| **This Chalet Chicken, Nutty Napa Slaw & Sweet Potato Wedges**<br><br>4 oz This Chalet Chicken (without skin), p. 131<br><br>1 cup Nutty Napa Slaw, p. 107<br><br>1 cup Sweet Potato Wedges, p. 116<br><br>*consider roasting 2 chickens and slicing and freezing the second for future meals | Choose 2 Cleanstart snacks (or more, if you're really hungry) from the list at the end of this meal plan (p. 48). | Do you need hummus? Salad dressing? Soup? Hard-boiled eggs? Today's the day to get ahead by making a batch of each in advance. |

# CHAPTER 8

# Week 1 Meal Plan

## Before you start the week, make:

- Easy Hummus, p. 145
- Beat the Band Balsamic, p. 142
- Consider premaking and freezing Lively Lentil Loaf, p. 125, and Lemony Fish Cakes, p. 124, if your Day 1 is busy

## Preparing for the week

I encourage you to go through the meal plan and recipes carefully, using this list and the Staples List as tools to determine what you already have and what you still need to make this week a success. If you are cooking for more than one, you will need to increase amounts for accompaniments like salads and rice as well as snacks. The lunch and dinner recipes generally serve a family, but where a separate protein is called for (such as chicken, fish and/or tofu), you will also need to scale amounts for your group.

# Grocery list of additional items

Please refer to the pantry, fridge and freezer staples list (pages 170–180) for weekly basics

- ○ 1 large container salad greens (any type)
- ○ 1 large container spinach
- ○ 1 bunch curly or flat-leafed kale
- ○ 2 garlic bulbs
- ○ 4 limes
- ○ 2 lemons
- ○ 1 avocado
- ○ 1 bunch green onions
- ○ 1 bunch fresh parsley
- ○ 1 bunch fresh cilantro
- ○ 1/4 cup fresh basil
- ○ fresh rosemary (optional)
- ○ 4 white potatoes
- ○ 4 sweet potatoes
- ○ 3 medium beets
- ○ 2 cups brussels sprouts
- ○ 1 cup fresh or frozen strawberries
- ○ 1 large bag frozen berries, any type
- ○ 1 cup frozen corn (choose organic to avoid GMO)
- ○ 3 yellow onions
- ○ 2 red onions
- ○ 3 shallots
- ○ 1 cabbage, any type
- ○ 8 oz white mushrooms
- ○ 1 apple (and more for snacks)
- ○ 2 oranges (and more for snacks)
- ○ 1 bag carrots
- ○ 1 bunch celery
- ○ 3 bell peppers, any combination of red, yellow and orange
- ○ additional veggies for pizza: olives, artichokes, mushrooms, bell pepper, tomato
- ○ additional veggies for stir-fry: broccoli, bok choy, bell peppers, mushrooms

- ○ 3 to 6 boneless chicken breasts (optional, you may choose tofu instead for Stir It Up!)
- ○ 454 g extra-lean ground turkey or chicken
- ○ 450 g white fish (fresh or frozen)
- ○ 1 block (454 g) firm or extra-firm tofu (optional, you may choose chicken instead for Stir It Up!)
- ○ 1 bag steel-cut oats (buy a bag, they will keep in your pantry)
- ○ 1 can (14 oz/398 mL) chickpeas
- ○ 3 cans (each 14 oz/398 mL) black beans
- ○ 1 can (14 oz/398 mL) kidney beans
- ○ 1 can (14 oz/398 mL) white beans
- ○ 2 cans (each 28 oz/798 mL) diced tomatoes
- ○ 1 can (28 oz/798 mL) crushed tomatoes
- ○ 1 can (28 oz/798 mL) whole tomatoes
- ○ 1 jar (28 oz/798 mL) natural tomato sauce or pasta sauce (no sugar added)
- ○ 2 tsp yellow mustard
- ○ 1 bag (450 g) green lentils
- ○ 1/4 cup raisins
- ○ 2 cups spelt flour
- ○ 2 1/4 cups whole wheat flour
- ○ quick rise or instant yeast
- ○ 1 L unsweetened almond milk
- ○ 1 L low-sodium vegetable broth
- ○ plain Greek yoghurt (for garnish)
- ○ 1 cup white cheddar, mozzarella or feta cheese
- ○ 1/4 cup (or more) grated Parmesan or Asiago cheese
- ○ 1 dozen eggs
- ○ 5 to 6 whole grain tortillas (if not making Wholly Homemade Tortillas)

| | Breakfast | Lunch | |
|---|---|---|---|
| 1 | **Cinnamon Oats & Berries** <br><br> 1 serving Cinnamon Oats & Berries, p. 86 <br><br> coffee or tea (with cow's milk or unsweetened dairy alternative; sweeten with a little honey, maple syrup or stevia, if necessary) | **The Big Salad:** 2 cups salad greens; 1/2 cup chopped grilled chicken, fish, tofu or beans of choice; 1 cup chopped raw veggies; 1 tsp sunflower or pumpkin seeds; 2 tbsp Beat the Band Balsamic, p. 142 <br><br> 1 piece fruit | |
| 2 | **Mason Jar Mornings** <br><br> 1 serving Mason Jar Mornings (p. 92); add fruit just before serving <br><br> coffee or tea (with cow's milk or unsweetened dairy alternative; sweeten with a little honey, maple syrup or stevia, if necessary) | **Lemony Fish Cake with Side Salad** <br><br> 1 Lemony Fish Cake, p. 124 <br><br> with side salad: 1 cup greens, 1 cup raw veggies of choice, 1 tbsp Beat the Band Balsamic, p. 142 <br><br> 1 piece of fruit | |
| 3 | **Eggs with Sautéed Greens & Avocado** <br><br> 1 serving Eggs with Sautéed Greens & Avocado, p. 87 <br><br> coffee or tea (with cow's milk or unsweetened dairy alternative; sweeten with a little honey, maple syrup or stevia, if necessary) | **Stir It Up!** <br><br> 1 serving of Stir It Up! with Nutty Lime or Simple Stir-fry Sauce, p. 139 <br><br> served over 1/2 cup brown rice or quinoa | |

| Dinner | Snacks | Evening Prep |
|---|---|---|
| **Lemony Fish Cakes with Rice & Oven-Roasted Veggies**<br><br>1 Lemony Fish Cake, p. 124<br><br>1 cup Oven-Roasted Veggies, p. 115<br><br>1/2 cup brown rice with 1/2 tsp butter or a squirt of low-sodium tamari or soy sauce<br><br>*set aside 1 Fish Cake for tomorrow's lunch | Choose 2 snacks daily from the Snack List, p. 82. | Assemble Mason Jar Mornings (p. 92) for tomorrow's breakfast and refrigerate overnight to allow it to soak. |
| **Stir It Up!**<br><br>1 serving of Stir It Up! with Nutty Lime or Simple Stir-fry Sauce, p. 139<br><br>served over 1/2 cup brown rice or quinoa<br><br>*make extra rice or quinoa and set aside 1 serving of Stir It Up & 1/2 cup rice or quinoa for tomorrow's lunch | Choose 2 snacks daily from the Snack List, p. 82. | If tomorrow night is busy, consider premaking Sopa Negro, p. 102, and/or Sweet P Biscuits, p. 146. |
| **Sopa Negro, Sweet P Biscuits & Sunshine Slaw**<br><br>1 cup Sopa Negro, p. 102<br><br>1 Sweet P Biscuit, p. 146<br><br>1 cup Sunshine Slaw, p. 108<br><br>*set aside 1 serving each of soup and biscuits and 1/2 cup slaw for tomorrow's lunch | Choose 2 snacks daily from the Snack List, p. 82. | Tomorrow's dinner, Crockpot Chicken Fajitas (p. 134) will cook in the crockpot while you're out, so get your veggies prepped tonight so you can quickly load the crockpot before you leave in the morning. If tomorrow night is busy, premake Wholly Homemade Tortillas (p. 147) and warm them slightly before serving with dinner. |

| | Breakfast | Lunch | |
|---|---|---|---|
| 4 | **Cinnamon Oats & Berries**<br><br>1 serving Cinnamon Oats & Berries, p. 86<br><br>coffee or tea (with cow's milk or unsweetened dairy alternative; sweeten with a little honey, maple syrup or stevia, if necessary) | **Sopa Negro & Sweet P Biscuit & Sunshine Slaw**<br><br>1 cup Sopa Negro, p. 102<br><br>1 Sweet P Biscuit, p. 146<br><br>1/2 cup Sunshine Slaw, p. 108 | |
| 5 | **Mason Jar Mornings**<br><br>1 serving Mason Jar Mornings (p. 92); add fruit just before serving<br><br>coffee or tea (with cow's milk or unsweetened dairy alternative; sweeten with a little honey, maple syrup or stevia, if necessary) | **Crockpot Chicken Fajitas**<br><br>1/2 cup shredded Crockpot Chicken, p. 134<br><br>1 cup cooked crockpot veggies<br><br>served over 1/2 cup brown rice or in 1 Wholly Homemade Tortilla (p. 147) topped with a dollop of plain Greek yoghurt and fresh chopped cilantro<br><br>1 piece of fruit or 1/2 cup berries | |
| 6 | **Eggs with Sautéed Greens & Avocado**<br><br>1 serving Eggs with Sautéed Greens & Avocado, p. 87<br><br>coffee or tea (with cow's milk or unsweetened dairy alternative; sweeten with a little honey, maple syrup or stevia, if necessary) | **Lively Lentil Loaf & Side Salad**<br><br>1 serving Lively Lentil Loaf, p. 125<br><br>with side salad: 1 cup greens, 1 cup raw veggies of choice, 1 tbsp Beat the Band Balsamic, p. 142 | |

| Dinner | Snacks | Evening Prep |
|---|---|---|
| **Crockpot Chicken Fajitas**<br><br>1/2 cup shredded Crockpot Chicken, p. 134<br><br>1 cup cooked crockpot veggies<br><br>served over 1/2 cup brown rice or in one Wholly Homemade Tortilla (p. 147) topped with a dollop of plain Greek yoghurt & fresh chopped cilantro.<br><br>with side salad: 1 cup greens, 1 cup raw veggies of choice, 1 tbsp Beat the Band Balsamic, p. 142<br><br>*set aside leftovers, including 1/2 cup rice, for tomorrow's lunch | Choose 2 snacks daily from the Snack List, p. 82. | Assemble Mason Jar Mornings (p. 92) for tomorrow's breakfast and refrigerate overnight to allow it to soak. |
| **Lively Lentil Loaf & Side Salad**<br><br>1 serving Lively Lentil Loaf, p. 125<br><br>with side salad: 1 cup greens, 1 cup raw veggies of choice, 1 tbsp Beat the Band Balsamic, p. 142<br><br>*set aside 1 serving of Lively Lentil Loaf for tomorrow's lunch | Choose 2 snacks daily from the Snack List, p. 82. | |
| **Easy Spelt Veggie Pizza and Last-Minute Lemony Kale Salad**<br><br>1 serving Easy Spelt Veggie Pizza, p. 140<br><br>1 cup Last-Minute Lemony Kale Salad, p. 111<br><br>*set aside 2 cups salad for tomorrow's lunch | Choose 2 snacks daily from the Snack List, p. 82. | Do you need soup for tomorrow's lunch or next week? Make a batch of Lemon-Basil Tomato Soup, p. 98, tonight if tomorrow is busy<br><br>Hard boil an egg for tomorrow's salad |

| | Breakfast | Lunch | |
|---|---|---|---|
| 7 | **Cinnamon Oats & Berries**<br><br>1 serving Cinnamon Oats & Berries, p. 86<br><br>coffee or tea (with cow's milk or unsweetened dairy alternative; sweeten with a little honey, maple syrup or stevia, if necessary) | **Lemon-Basil Tomato Soup & Last-Minute Lemony Kale Salad**<br><br>1 cup Lemon-Basil Tomato Soup, p. 98<br><br>2 cups leftover Last-Minute Lemony Kale Salad, p. 111, with a hard-boiled egg sliced on top or on the side | |

| Dinner | Snacks | Evening Prep |
|---|---|---|
| **Santa Fe Turkey Chili**<br><br>1 cup Santa Fe Turkey Chili (meat-free option in recipe), p. 123, topped with 1 to 2 tbsp plain Greek yoghurt<br><br>served over 1/2 cup brown rice or quinoa | Choose 2 snacks daily from the Snack List, p. 82. | Do you need hummus? Salad dressing? Soup? Hard-boiled eggs? Today's the day to get ahead by making a batch of each in advance. |

# CHAPTER 9

# Week 2 Meal Plan

## Before you start the week, make:

- Easy Hummus, p. 145
- Berry Balsamic, p. 142
- Consider premaking and refrigerating Beta Butternut Soup, p. 100
- Consider premaking and refrigerating Salsa Burgers, p. 117

## Preparing for the week

I encourage you to go through the meal plan and recipes carefully, using this list and the Staples List as tools to determine what you already have and what you still need to make this week a success. If you are cooking for more than one, you will need to increase amounts for accompaniments like salads and rice as well as snacks. The lunch and dinner recipes generally serve a family, but where a separate protein is called for (such as chicken, fish and/or tofu), you will also need to scale amounts for your group.

## Grocery list of additional items

Please refer to the pantry, fridge and freezer staples list (pages 170–180) for
weekly basics

- 1 large container spinach
- 1 large container salad greens
- 2 large bunches curly or flat-leafed kale
- 6 yellow onions
- 2 red onions
- 2 to 3 garlic bulbs
- 4 sweet potatoes or yams
- 2 white potatoes
- 1 bag carrots
- 1 bunch celery
- 1 green bell pepper
- 1 cucumber
- 2 to 3 tomatoes
- 6 medium beets
- 4 cups brussels sprouts
- 1 butternut squash
- 1 spaghetti squash
- 1 or more portobello mushroom caps (enough for your family)
- additional veggies for pizza: olives, artichokes, mushrooms, bell pepper, tomato
- 1 bunch fresh cilantro
- fresh rosemary (optional)
- fresh sage (optional)
- 2 cups fresh or frozen strawberries
- 1 bag frozen berries, any type
- 1 avocado
- 1 bunch bananas
- 1 bag apples, pears or oranges for snacks
- 3 lemons
- 1 lime
- 2 lb (0.9 kg) ground turkey, pork, chicken or lean beef
- 1 lb (454 g) lean ground beef
- 6 or more chicken breasts (depending on how often you will be opting for chicken)
- 1 fresh or frozen white fish fillet (optional)
- 1 block (454 g) firm organic tofu (optional)
- 2 cans (each 14 oz/398 mL) chickpeas
- 2 cans (each 14 oz/398 mL) black beans
- 1 can (14 oz/398 mL) kidney beans
- 1 can (28 oz/798 mL) diced tomatoes
- 1 can (28 oz/798 mL) crushed tomatoes
- 1 can (28 oz/798 mL) whole tomatoes
- 1 jar (28 oz/798 mL) natural tomato sauce or pasta sauce (no sugar added)
- 2 cups spelt flour
- 1 1/2 tsp quick-rising or instant yeast
- 1/2 cup raw cashews
- 1 1/2 cups 100% whole grain macaroni noodles
- 1 1/2 cups grated Parmesan or Asiago cheese
- 1/2 cup feta cheese
- 1 container (500g) plain Greek yoghurt
- 1 1/2 cups shredded white cheddar cheese
- 1 loaf Ezekiel sprouted grain bread (optional, buy and store in freezer)
- 1 L low-sodium vegetable broth
- 1 L unsweetened almond milk
- 1 dozen eggs (or more)

| | Breakfast | Lunch | |
|---|---|---|---|
| 1 | **Take It to Go!**<br><br>2 hard-boiled eggs<br><br>1 piece fruit or 1 cup berries<br><br>coffee or tea (with cow's milk or unsweetened dairy alternative; sweeten with a little honey, maple syrup or stevia, if necessary) | **The Big Salad:** 2 cups salad greens; 1/2 cup chopped grilled chicken, fish, tofu or beans of choice; 1 cup chopped raw veggies; 1 tsp sunflower or pumpkin seeds; 2 tbsp Berry Balsamic, p. 142<br><br>1 piece fruit of choice | |
| 2 | **Cinnamon Oats & Berries**<br><br>1 serving Cinnamon Oats & Berries, p. 86<br><br>coffee or tea (with cow's milk or unsweetened dairy alternative; sweeten with a little honey, maple syrup or stevia, if necessary) | **Salsa Burgers & Zesty Kale Caesar Salad**<br><br>1 Salsa Burger, p. 117 (or veggie burger of choice), no bun<br><br>served with 1 1/2 cups Zesty Kale Salad, p. 113 (no croutons)<br><br>*set aside 1 burger and 1 1/2 cups salad for tomorrow's lunch | |
| 3 | **PB & J Breakfast Smoothie**<br><br>1 serving PB & J Breakfast Smoothie, p. 94<br><br>coffee or tea (with cow's milk or unsweetened dairy alternative; sweeten with a little honey, maple syrup or stevia, if necessary) | **Beta Butternut Soup & Big Salad**<br><br>1 cup Beta Butternut Soup, p. 100<br><br>with a Big Salad: 2 cups greens; 1/2 cup chopped cooked chicken, tofu or beans of choice; 1 cup chopped raw veggies of choice; 2 tbsp Berry Balsamic, p. 142 | |

| Dinner | Snacks | Evening Prep |
|---|---|---|
| **Salsa Burgers & Zesty Kale Caesar Salad**<br><br>1 Salsa Burger, p. 117 (or veggie burger of choice, see Mains, pp. 117–121), no bun or served in half a small whole wheat pita with sliced tomato and greens<br><br>served with 1 1/2 cups Zesty Kale Salad, p 111 (no croutons)<br><br>*set aside 1 burger and 1 1/2 cups salad for tomorrow's lunch | Choose 2 snacks daily from the Snack List, p. 82. | |
| **Grilled Chicken, Fish or Tofu with Grilled Veggies and Salad**<br><br>4 oz chicken or fish or 1/4 of a 454 g block of organic tofu, brushed with a little olive oil and garlic and grilled or pan-fried<br><br>1 cup Oven-Roasted Veggies, p. 115<br><br>with side salad: 1 cup greens, 1/2 to 1 cup chopped raw veggies of choice and 1 tbsp Berry Balsamic, p. 142 | Choose 2 snacks daily from the Snack List, p. 82. | Make Beta Butternut Soup (p. 100) for tomorrow's lunch if you did not premake it on the weekend. |
| **Mexican Spaghetti Squash Bake & Side Salad**<br><br>1 serving Mexican Spaghetti Squash Bake, p. 136<br><br>with side salad: 1 cup greens, 1/2 to 1 cup chopped raw veggies of choice and 1 tbsp Berry Balsamic, p. 142<br><br>1 piece of fruit<br><br>*set aside 1 serving Mexican Spaghetti Squash Bake for tomorrow's lunch | Choose 2 snacks daily from the Snack List, p. 82. | Mama's Little Helper (p. 135) will cook in the crockpot while you are out tomorrow. Pre-browning your ground beef and chopping your veggies tonight will allow you to toss them in the crockpot quickly in the morning. |

| | Breakfast | Lunch | |
|---|---|---|---|
| **4** | **Eggs with Sautéed Greens & Avocado**<br><br>1 serving Eggs with Sautéed Greens & Avocado, p. 87<br><br>coffee or tea (with cow's milk or unsweetened dairy alternative; sweeten with a little honey, maple syrup or stevia, if necessary) | **Mexican Spaghetti Squash Bake**<br><br>1 serving leftover Mexican Spaghetti Squash Bake, p. 136<br><br>1 brown rice cake or 1/2 small whole wheat pita with 1 tsp natural peanut or almond butter<br><br>1 piece fruit or 1 cup berries | |
| **5** | **Cinnamon Oats & Berries**<br><br>1 serving Cinnamon Oats & Berries, p. 86<br><br>coffee or tea (with cow's milk or unsweetened dairy alternative; sweeten with a little honey, maple syrup or stevia, if necessary) | **Mama's Little Helper & Side Salad**<br><br>1 cup leftover Mama's Little Helper, p. 135<br><br>with side salad: 1 cup greens, 1/2 to 1 cup chopped raw veggies of choice and 1 tbsp Berry Balsamic, p. 142 | |
| **6** | **Portobello Eggs Benny with Cashew Hollandaise**<br><br>1 serving of Portobello Eggs Benny, p. 90<br><br>1 piece fruit or 1 cup berries<br><br>coffee or tea (with cow's milk or unsweetened dairy alternative; sweeten with a little honey, maple syrup or stevia, if necessary)<br><br>*set aside leftover Cashew Hollandaise for tomorrow's breakfast | **Simple Chili over Brown Rice**<br><br>1 cup Simple Chili, p. 119<br><br>served over 1/2 cup brown rice<br><br>1 piece fruit | |
| **7** | **Poached Egg on Toast with Cashew Hollandaise**<br><br>1 poached egg and<br><br>1 cup spinach, sautéed<br><br>served on 1 slice sprouted or 100% whole grain bread<br><br>topped with 1 to 2 tbsp Cashew Hollandaise, p. 90<br><br>coffee or tea (with cow's milk or unsweetened dairy alternative; sweeten with a little honey, maple syrup or stevia, if necessary) | **Beta Butternut Soup or Simple Chili & Last-Minute Lemony Kale Salad**<br><br>1 cup Beta Butternut Soup (p. 100) or 1 cup Simple Chili, p. 119<br><br>1 1/2 cups Last-Minute Lemony Kale Salad, p. 111 1 brown rice cake or 1/2 small whole wheat pita with 1 tsp natural peanut or almond butter | |

| Dinner | Snacks | Evening Prep |
|---|---|---|
| **Mama's Little Helper & Side Salad**<br><br>1 1/2 cups Mama's Little Helper, p. 135<br><br>with side salad: 1 cup greens, 1/2 to 1 cup chopped raw veggies of choice and 1 tbsp Berry Balsamic, p. 142<br><br>*set aside 1 cup Mama's Little Helper for tomorrow's lunch | Choose 2 snacks daily from the Snack List, p. 82. | Tomorrow night's Simple Chili (p. 119) can be cooked in a crockpot, so if tomorrow is busy, prepare your veggies today. Tomorrow morning, put them in the crockpot raw and cook on low for 8 hours. |
| **Simple Chili over Brown Rice**<br><br>1 cup Simple Chili (p. 119) garnished with 2 tbsp plain Greek yoghurt (optional)<br><br>served over 1/2 cup brown rice<br><br>with raw veggies or side salad: 1 cup greens, 1/2 to 1 cup chopped raw veggies of choice and 1 tbsp Berry Balsamic, p. 142 | Choose 2 snacks daily from the Snack List, p. 82. | |
| **Easy Spelt Veggie Pizza & Last-Minute Lemony Kale Salad**<br><br>**1 serving Easy Spelt Veggie Pizza, p. 140**<br><br>**1 cup Last-Minute Lemony Kale Salad, p. 111** | Choose 2 snacks daily from the Snack List, p. 82. | |
| **Maple-Sage Roasted Chicken Dinner & Side Salad**<br><br>1 serving Maple-Sage Roasted Chicken Dinner, p. 128<br><br>with a side salad: 1 cup greens, 1/2 to 1 cup chopped raw veggies of choice and 1 tbsp Berry Balsamic, p. 142 | Choose 2 snacks daily from the Snack List, p. 82. | Do you need hummus? Salad dressing? Soup? Hard-boiled eggs? Today's the day to get ahead by making a batch of each in advance. |

# CHAPTER 10

# Week 3 Meal Plan

## Before you start the week, make:

- Easy Hummus, p. 145
- Green Goddess Dressing, p. 143
- Consider premaking and refrigerating Thai This Soup, p. 101

## Preparing for the week

I encourage you to go through the meal plan and recipes carefully, using this list and the Staples List as tools to determine what you already have and what you still need to make this week a success. If you are cooking for more than one, you will need to increase amounts for accompaniments like salads and rice as well as snacks. The lunch and dinner recipes generally serve a family, but where a separate protein is called for (such as chicken, fish and/or tofu), you will also need to scale amounts for your group.

## Grocery list of additional items

Please refer to the pantry, fridge and freezer staples list (pages 170–180) for weekly basics

- 1 large container spinach
- 1 large container salad greens
- 1 large bunch curly or flat-leafed kale
- 4 yellow onions
- 1 red onion
- 2 garlic bulbs
- 4 sweet potatoes or yams
- 1 bag white potatoes
- 1.5 lb baby potatoes (or equivalent in large white potatoes)
- 1 bag carrots
- 1 bunch celery
- 20 oz white mushrooms
- 2 green bell peppers
- 1 cup fresh or frozen green peas
- 2 heads broccoli
- 2 medium or 4 small zucchini
- 1 napa cabbage
- 1 small purple cabbage
- 1 cucumber
- 6 medium tomatoes
- 16 oz grape tomatoes
- 1 cup alfalfa sprouts (optional)
- 1 bunch fresh cilantro
- 1 bunch fresh parsley 1 cup fresh basil
- fresh rosemary (optional)
- 1 1/2 tbsp fresh tarragon
- 1 tbsp fresh chives (or 1 tsp dried)
- 1 ginger root
- 1 bag frozen berries, any type
- 2 avocados
- 3 lemons
- 3 limes
- apples, pears, bananas and/or oranges for snacks

- 6 or more chicken breasts (depending on how often you will be opting for chicken)
- 1 to 3 fresh or frozen white fish fillets (optional)
- 2 blocks (each 454 g) firm organic tofu (optional)
- 2 cans (each 14 oz/398 mL) chickpeas
- 1 can (28 oz/798 mL) crushed tomatoes
- 1 can (28 oz/798 mL) whole tomatoes
- 1 can (400 mL) coconut milk
- 2 tsp red wine vinegar
- 1/4 cup raw cashews or peanuts
- 1/2 cup chopped walnuts
- 1 tbsp capers or 1 large dill pickle
- 1 small jar red curry (or harissa) paste
- 1 bag (450 g) green lentils or 1 can (14 oz/398 mL) green lentils
- 1 bag (450g) yellow split peas
- 2 bags (each 454 g) 100% whole grain pasta (penne or rotini)
- 1/2 cup grated Parmesan or Asiago cheese
- 1 container (500g) plain Greek yoghurt
- 1 loaf Ezekiel sprouted grain bread (optional, buy and store in freezer)
- 6 small whole grain pitas
- 1 L low-sodium vegetable broth
- 2 L low-sodium chicken broth
- 1 L unsweetened almond milk
- 1 dozen eggs (or more)

|   | **Breakfast** | **Lunch** |   |
|---|---|---|---|
| **1** | **The Breakfast Salad**<br><br>1 serving Breakfast Salad, p. 97<br><br>coffee or tea (with cow's milk or unsweetened dairy alternative; sweeten with a little honey, maple syrup or stevia, if necessary) | **Hummus & Veggie Pita with Soup or Fruit**<br><br>1/2 small whole wheat pita filled with 2 tbsp Easy Hummus (p. 145) and some or all of: sliced cucumber, tomato, bell pepper, sprouts and spinach or other green leafy veggie<br><br>1 cup soup of choice (from Soups, Salads & Sides, pp. 98–104)<br><br>or 1 piece fruit |   |
| **2** | **Cinnamon Oats & Berries**<br><br>1 serving Cinnamon Oats & Berries, p. 86<br><br>coffee or tea (with cow's milk or unsweetened dairy alternative; sweeten with a little honey, maple syrup or stevia, if necessary) | **Thai This Soup, Sweet P Biscuit & Nutty Napa Slaw**<br><br>1 cup Thai This Soup, p. 101<br><br>1 Sweet P Biscuit, p. 146<br><br>1 cup Nutty Napa Slaw, p. 107 |   |
| **3** | **Avocado Egg Toast**<br><br>1 serving Avocado Egg Toast, p. 94<br><br>coffee or tea (with cow's milk or unsweetened dairy alternative; sweeten with a little honey, maple syrup or stevia, if necessary) | **Smashed Chickpea Salad Pita**<br><br>2/3 cup Smashed Chickpea Salad (p. 111) served in 1/2 small whole wheat pita with sliced tomato, spinach and sprouts<br><br>1 piece fruit of choice<br><br>*set aside 2/3 cup Smashed Chickpea Salad for tomorrow's lunch |   |

| Dinner | Snacks | Evening Prep |
|---|---|---|
| **Thai This Soup, Sweet P Biscuits & Nutty Napa Slaw**<br><br>1 1/2 cups Thai This Soup, p. 101<br><br>1 Sweet P Biscuit, p. 146<br><br>1 cup Nutty Napa Slaw, p. 107<br><br>*set aside 1 cup Thai This Soup, 1 Sweet P Biscuit & 1 cup Nutty Napa Slaw for tomorrow's lunch<br><br>*Freeze rest of Sweet P Biscuits for Day 5 dinner | Choose 2 snacks daily from the Snack List, p. 82. | |
| **Grilled Chicken, Fish or Tofu with Sweet Potato Wedges & Side Salad**<br><br>4 oz of chicken or fish or 1/5 of 454 g block of organic tofu, brushed with a little olive oil and garlic then grilled or pan-fried<br><br>1 cup Sweet Potato Wedges, p. 116<br><br>with side salad: 1 cup greens, 1/2 to 1 cup chopped raw veggies of choice and 1 tbsp Green Goddess Dressing, p. 143 | Choose 2 snacks daily from the Snack List, p. 82. | Make Smashed Chickpea Salad (p. 111) for tomorrow's lunch. |
| **Zucchini Noodles with Avocado Pesto**<br><br>2 1/2 cups raw zucchini noodles served with 2 tbsp Avocado Pesto, p. 137<br><br>top with 4 oz grilled chicken breast or 1/4 of 454 g block of firm organic tofu, grilled or sautéed in 1 tsp coconut oil | Choose 2 snacks daily from the Snack List, p. 82. | If tomorrow night is busy, pre-cook the lentils and prepare the veggies for tomorrow's Lentil Sloppy Joes (p. 133) and refrigerate |

| | Breakfast | Lunch | |
|---|---|---|---|
| 4 | **Eggs with Sautéed Greens & Avocado**<br><br>1 serving Eggs with Sautéed Greens & Avocado, p. 87<br><br>coffee or tea (with cow's milk or unsweetened dairy alternative; sweeten with a little honey, maple syrup or stevia, if necessary) | **Smashed Chickpea Salad Pita**<br><br>2/3 cup Smashed Chickpea Salad (p. 111) served in 1/2 small whole wheat pita with sliced tomato, spinach and sprouts<br><br>1 piece fruit of choice | |
| 5 | **Cinnamon Oats & Berries**<br><br>1 serving Cinnamon Oats & Berries, p. 86<br><br>coffee or tea (with cow's milk or unsweetened dairy alternative; sweeten with a little honey, maple syrup or stevia, if necessary) | **Lentil Sloppy Joes**<br><br>3/4 cup Sloppy Joe mixture (p. 133) served over 1 slice of toasted Ezekiel sprouted grain bread<br><br>top with 1 tbsp grated Asiago or Parmesan (optional)<br><br>1 piece of fruit | |
| 6 | **Avocado Egg Toast**<br><br>1 serving Avocado Egg Toast, p. 94<br><br>coffee or tea (with cow's milk or unsweetened dairy alternative; sweeten with a little honey, maple syrup or stevia, if necessary) | **Mexican Chicken Soup & Sweet P Biscuits**<br><br>1 1/2 cups Mexican Chicken Soup, p. 104<br><br>1 Sweet P Biscuit, p. 146 | |
| 7 | **The Breakfast Salad**<br><br>1 serving Breakfast Salad, p. 97<br><br>coffee or tea (with cow's milk or unsweetened dairy alternative; sweeten with a little honey, maple syrup or stevia, if necessary) | **Warm Gribiche Salad**<br><br>2 cups Warm Gribiche Salad, p. 114<br><br>or 1 cup leftover Warm Gribiche Salad and 4 oz. chicken breast, piece of white fish or 1/4 of 454 g block of organic tofu, grilled or baked | |

| Dinner | Snacks | Evening Prep |
|---|---|---|
| **Lentil Sloppy Joes**<br><br>3/4 cup Sloppy Joe mixture (p. 133) served over 2 slices toasted Ezekiel sprouted grain bread<br><br>top with 2 tbsp grated Asiago or Parmesan (optional)<br><br>1 cup raw or cooked broccoli<br><br>*set aside 1 serving of Sloppy Joe mixture for tomorrow's lunch | Choose 2 snacks daily from the Snack List, p. 82. | |
| **Mexican Chicken Soup & Sweet P Biscuits**<br><br>1 1/2 cups Mexican Chicken Soup, p. 104<br><br>1 Sweet P Biscuit, p. 146<br><br>1 piece of fruit<br><br>or side salad: 1 cup greens, 1/2 to 1 cup chopped raw veggies of choice and 1 tbsp Green Goddess Dressing, p. 143<br><br>*set aside 1 serving of soup and 1 biscuit for tomorrow's lunch | Choose 2 snacks daily from the Snack List, p. 82. | |
| **Warm Gribiche Salad with Grilled Chicken, Fish or Tofu**<br><br>4 oz chicken breast, piece of white fish or 1/4 of 454 g block of organic tofu, grilled or baked<br><br>1 cup Warm Gribiche Salad, p. 114<br><br>*set aside 2 cups Warm Gribiche Salad for tomorrow's lunch | Choose 2 snacks daily from the Snack List, p. 82. | |
| **Shepherd's Pie with Rosemary Mashed Potatoes & Side Salad**<br><br>1 serving Shepherd's Pie with Rosemary Mashed Potatoes, p. 129<br><br>with side salad: 1 cup greens, 1/2 to 1 cup chopped raw veggies of choice and 1 tbsp Green Goddess Dressing, p. 143 | Choose 2 snacks daily from the Snack List, p. 82. | Do you need hummus? Salad dressing? Soup? Hard-boiled eggs? Today's the day to get ahead by making a batch of each in advance. |

# CHAPTER 11

# Week 4 Meal Plan

## Before you start the week, make:

- Easy Hummus, p. 145
- Sesame-Maple Vinaigrette, p. 143
- Dillicious French Lentil Salad, p. 112
- Roasted Red Pepper & Kale Egg Cups, p. 89
- Consider premaking (or at least cooking/prepping lentils and veggies) Buddha Burgers, p. 118

## Preparing for the week

I encourage you to go through the meal plan and recipes carefully, using this list and the Staples List as tools to determine what you already have and what you still need to make this week a success. If you are cooking for more than one, you will need to increase amounts for accompaniments like salads and rice as well as snacks. The lunch and dinner recipes generally serve a family, but where a separate protein is called for (such as chicken, fish and/or tofu), you will also need to scale amounts for your group.

# Grocery list of additional items

Please refer to the pantry, fridge and freezer staples list (pages 170–180) for weekly basics

- 1 large container spinach
- 1 large container salad greens
- 3 large bunches curly or flat-leafed kale
- 3 yellow onions
- 2 red onions
- 2 bunches green onions
- 2 garlic bulbs
- 1 sweet potato
- 1 bag carrots
- 1 bunch celery
- 16 oz white mushrooms
- 1 red bell pepper
- 1 cup fresh or frozen green peas
- 1 cup fresh or frozen corn (choose organic to avoid GMO)
- 1 small head broccoli
- 5 to 6 leeks
- 3 medium beets
- 1 zucchini
- 1 small cabbage, any type
- 1 to 2 cucumbers
- 4 to 5 medium tomatoes
- 1 bunch fresh cilantro
- 1 bunch fresh parsley
- 1 cup fresh basil
- fresh rosemary (optional)
- 1 package fresh tarragon
- 1 tbsp dill (or 1 tsp dried)
- 1 to 2 kg bag frozen berries, any type (for oatmeal)
- 2 avocados
- apples, pears, bananas and/or oranges for snacks
- 4 to 5 lemons
- 4 limes

- 3 or more chicken breasts (depending on how often you will be opting for chicken)
- 454 g frozen or fresh white fish fillets (optional, you may choose tofu instead for Taco Tuesdays)
- 3 blocks (each 454 g) firm organic tofu (1 to 2 blocks are optional; you may choose chicken instead for Taco Tuesdays and in Thai Rice Noodle Salad)
- 1 can (14 oz/398 mL) chickpeas
- 1 can (14 oz/398 mL) white beans
- 1 can (14 oz/398 mL) black beans
- 2 tbsp red wine vinegar
- 1 small jar roasted sweet red bell peppers (you need only 1/2 cup)
- 1/4 cup raw cashews or peanuts (optional)
- 1/2 cup raw almonds
- 3/4 cup dried green lentils
- 1 bag (450 g) red lentils
- 3/4 cup grated Parmesan or Asiago cheese
- 2 tbsp goat cheese (optional)
- 1 container (500g) plain Greek yoghurt
- 6 small whole grain pitas (optional)
- 1 package (454 g) rice noodles (vermicelli or thicker noodle)
- 1 L low-sodium chicken broth
- 2 L unsweetened almond milk
- 2 dozen eggs (or more)

| | Breakfast | Lunch | |
|---|---|---|---|
| **1** | **Roasted Red Pepper & Kale Egg Cups**<br><br>2 Roasted Red Pepper & Kale Egg Cups, p. 89<br><br>1 small piece fruit, half a banana or 1/2 cup berries<br><br>coffee or tea (with cow's milk or unsweetened dairy alternative; sweeten with a little honey, maple syrup or stevia, if necessary)<br><br>*refrigerate some Egg Cups for this week's breakfasts and freeze leftovers | **Dillicious French Lentil Salad**<br><br>1 cup Dillicious French Lentil Salad, p. 112<br><br>served over 1 cup salad greens<br><br>half a small whole wheat pita<br><br>*set aside 1 cup Lentil Salad and refrigerate for Day 3's lunch | |
| **2** | **Cinnamon Oats & Berries**<br><br>1 serving Cinnamon Oats & Berries, p. 86<br><br>coffee or tea (with cow's milk or unsweetened dairy alternative; sweeten with a little honey, maple syrup or stevia, if necessary) | **Buddha Burger with Zesty Kale Caesar Salad**<br><br>1 Buddha Burger (p. 118) topped with 1 tbsp Smoky Mayo, p. 144<br><br>served with 1 1/2 cups Zesty Kale Caesar Salad, p. 113 (no croutons) | |
| **3** | **Roasted Red Pepper & Kale Egg Cups**<br><br>2 Roasted Red Pepper & Kale Egg Cups, p. 89<br><br>1 small piece fruit, half a banana or 1/2 cup berries<br><br>coffee or tea (with cow's milk or unsweetened dairy alternative; sweeten with a little honey, maple syrup or stevia, if necessary) | **Dillicious French Lentil Salad**<br><br>1 cup Dillicious French Lentil Salad, p. 112<br><br>served over 1 cup salad greens<br><br>half small whole wheat pita | |

| Dinner | Snacks | Evening Prep |
|---|---|---|
| **Buddha Burgers with Zesty Kale Caesar Salad**<br><br>1 Buddha Burger (p. 118) topped with 1 tbsp Smoky Mayo, p. 144 (mayo optional)<br><br>served in half small whole wheat pita (optional)<br><br>served with 1 1/2 cups Zesty Kale Caesar Salad, p. 113 (no croutons)<br><br>*set aside 1 burger and 1 1/2 cups Zesty Kale Caesar for tomorrow's lunch | Choose 2 snacks daily from the Snack List, p. 82. | Premake a batch of Wholly Homemade Tortillas (p. 147) if using for tomorrow night's tacos. |
| **Taco Tuesday Two Ways & Side Salad**<br><br>1 serving Taco Tuesday Two Ways (your choice of fish or tofu filling), p. 138, using Wholly Homemade Tortillas (p. 147) or store-bought 100% whole grain tortillas<br><br>with side salad: 1 cup greens, 1/2 to 1 cup chopped raw veggies of choice and 1 tbsp Sesame-Maple Vinaigrette, p. 143 | Choose 2 snacks daily from the Snack List, p. 82. | |
| **Zucchini Pie with Tarragon Asiago Rice Crust & Last-Minute Lemony Kale Salad**<br><br>1 serving Zucchini Pie, p. 93<br><br>1 1/2 cups Last-Minute Lemony Kale Salad, p. 111<br><br>1 piece fruit or 1 cup berries<br><br>*set aside 1 serving of Zucchini Pie and 1 1/2 cups Kale Salad for tomorrow's lunch | Choose 2 snacks daily from the Snack List, p. 82. | Assemble Mason Jar Mornings (p. 92) for tomorrow's breakfast and refrigerate overnight to allow it to soak. |

| | Breakfast | Lunch | |
|---|---|---|---|
| 4 | **Mason Jar Mornings**<br><br>1 serving Mason Jar Mornings (p. 92); add fruit just before serving<br><br>coffee or tea (with cow's milk or unsweetened dairy alternative; sweeten with a little honey, maple syrup or stevia, if necessary) | **Zucchini Pie with Tarragon Asiago Rice Crust & Last-Minute Lemony Kale Salad**<br><br>1 serving Zucchini Pie, p. 93<br><br>1 1/2 cups Last-Minute Lemony Kale Salad, p. 111 | |
| 5 | **Eggs with Sautéed Greens & Avocado**<br><br>1 serving Eggs with Sautéed Greens & Avocado, p. 87<br><br>coffee or tea (with cow's milk or unsweetened dairy alternative; sweeten with a little honey, maple syrup or stevia, if necessary) | **Syrian Lentil Soup with Sweet P Biscuit**<br><br>1 1/2 cups Syrian Lentil Soup, p. 103<br><br>1 Sweet P Biscuit, p. 146 | |
| 6 | **Cinnamon Oats & Berries**<br><br>1 serving Cinnamon Oats & Berries, p. 86<br><br>coffee or tea (with cow's milk or unsweetened dairy alternative; sweeten with a little honey, maple syrup or stevia, if necessary) | **Thai Rice Noodle Salad**<br><br>1 1/2 cups Thai Rice Noodle Salad, p. 109 | |
| 7 | **Anytime Tofu Scramble**<br><br>1 serving Anytime Tofu Scramble, p. 88<br><br>1 piece sprouted grain or 100% whole grain bread toasted with 1/2 tsp butter<br><br>coffee or tea (with cow's milk or unsweetened dairy alternative; sweeten with a little honey, maple syrup or stevia, if necessary) | **Cancun Quinoa**<br><br>1 cup Cancun Quinoa, p. 105<br><br>1 fruit or 1 cup berries | |

| Dinner | Snacks | Evening Prep |
|---|---|---|
| **Syrian Lentil Soup with Sweet P Biscuits**<br><br>1 1/2 cups Syrian Lentil Soup, p. 103<br><br>1 Sweet P Biscuit, p. 146<br><br>serve with raw veggies (optional)<br><br>*set aside 1 1/2 cups Lentil Soup and 1 biscuit for tomorrow's lunch | Choose 2 snacks daily from the Snack List, p. 82. | |
| **Thai Rice Noodle Salad**<br><br>1 1/2 cups Thai Rice Noodle Salad, p. 109<br><br>1 small piece of fruit, half a banana or 1/2 cup fruit<br><br>*set aside 1 1/2 cups of Thai Rice Noodle Salad for tomorrow's lunch | Choose 2 snacks daily from the Snack List, p. 82. | |
| **Creamy Leeks & White Beans with Tarragon**<br><br>1 cup Creamy Leeks & White Beans with Tarragon, p. 126<br><br>served over 1/2 cup brown rice<br><br>with side salad: 1 cup greens, 1/2 to 1 cup chopped raw veggies of choice and 1 tbsp Sesame-Maple Vinaigrette, p. 143 | Choose 2 snacks daily from the Snack List, p. 82. | Pre-cook and refrigerate quinoa for tomorrow's lunch, Cancun Quinoa (p. 105) |
| **Bottomless Chicken Pot Pie & Side Salad**<br><br>1 serving Bottomless Chicken Pot Pie, p. 132<br><br>side of raw or cooked veggies of choice or side salad: 1 cup greens, 1/2 to 1 cup chopped raw veggies of choice and 1 tbsp Sesame-Maple Vinaigrette, p. 143 | Choose 2 snacks daily from the Snack List, p. 82. | Do you need hummus? Salad dressing? Soup? Hard-boiled eggs? Today's the day to get ahead by making a batch of each in advance. |

# CHAPTER 12

## Week 5 Meal Plan

### Before you start the week, make:

- Easy Hummus, p. 145
- Beat the Band Balsamic, p. 142
- Lemon-Basil Tomato Soup, p. 98
- Roasted Red Pepper & Kale Egg Cups, p. 89
- Consider premaking Don't Falafel the Wagon, p. 127
- Consider premaking and refrigerating or freezing Spicy Black Bean Burgers, p. 121

### Preparing for the week

I encourage you to go through the meal plan and recipes carefully, using this list and the Staples List as tools to determine what you already have and what you still need to make this week a success. If you are cooking for more than one, you will need to increase amounts for accompaniments like salads and rice as well as snacks. The lunch and dinner recipes generally serve a family, but where a separate protein is called for (such as chicken, fish and/or tofu), you will also need to scale amounts for your group.

# Grocery list of additional items

Please refer to the pantry, fridge and freezer staples list (pages 170–180) for weekly basics

- 1 large container spinach
- 1 large container salad greens
- 2 large bunches of curly or flat-leafed kale
- 1 bunch Tuscan (or lacinato) kale
- 2 yellow onions
- 4 shallots
- 1 bunch green onions
- 2 garlic bulbs
- 3 sweet potatoes
- 1 bag carrots
- 1 bunch celery
- 1 small purple cabbage
- 1 napa cabbage
- 1 butternut squash
- 2 leeks
- 1 cucumber
- 2 medium tomatoes
- 1 bunch fresh cilantro
- 1 bunch fresh parsley
- 1/3 cup fresh basil
- 1 fresh ginger root (unless you have some in your freezer)
- additional veggies for stir-fry: broccoli, bok choy, bell peppers, mushrooms
- 1 1/2 cups fresh or frozen strawberries
- 1 avocado
- 1 orange (and more for snacks)
- 1 banana (and more for snacks)
- apples and pears for snacks
- 4 lemons
- 3 limes
- 1 to 2 roasting chickens (2 if you are roasting one to use in later meals)

- 454 g lean ground beef (preferably grass-fed)
- 1 can (14 oz/398 mL) white beans
- 2 cans (each 14 oz/398 mL) chickpeas
- 1 can (14 oz/398 mL) black beans
- 1 can (28oz/798 mL) diced tomatoes
- 1 can (28 oz/798 mL) whole tomatoes
- 1/4 cup raw cashews or peanuts (optional)
- 1/4 cup sesame seeds (optional)
- 1/2 cup chopped walnuts
- 3/4 cup grated Parmesan or Asiago cheese
- 1/4 cup feta (optional)
- 1/3 cup shredded white cheddar cheese
- 1 container (500g) plain Greek yoghurt
- 1 1/2 cups dried 100% whole grain macaroni noodles
- 1 tsp poultry seasoning
- 1 loaf Ezekiel sprouted grain bread (store in freezer)
- 2 L low-sodium veggie broth
- 1 L unsweetened almond milk
- 1 dozen eggs (or more)

|   | Breakfast | Lunch |  |
|---|-----------|-------|---|
| **1** | **PB & J Breakfast Smoothie**<br><br>1 serving PB & J Breakfast Smoothie, p. 94<br><br>coffee or tea (with cow's milk or unsweetened dairy alternative; sweeten with a little honey, maple syrup or stevia, if necessary) | **Lemon-Basil Tomato Soup & Side Salad**<br><br>1 cup Lemon-Basil Tomato Soup, p. 98<br><br>with side salad: 1 cup greens, 1/2 to 1 cup chopped raw veggies of choice and 1 tbsp salad dressing of choice, pp. 141–143 |  |
| **2** | **Breakfast to Go!**<br><br>2 hard-boiled eggs<br><br>1 fruit or 1 cup berries<br><br>12 raw almonds<br><br>coffee or tea (with cow's milk or unsweetened dairy alternative; sweeten with a little honey, maple syrup or stevia, if necessary) | **Don't Falafel the Wagon & Last-Minute Lemony Kale Salad**<br><br>1 serving Don't Falafel the Wagon, p. 127<br><br>1 1/2 cups Last-Minute Lemony Kale Salad, p. 111 |  |
| **3** | **Cinnamon Oats & Berries**<br><br>1 serving Cinnamon Oats & Berries, p. 86<br><br>coffee or tea (with cow's milk or unsweetened dairy alternative; sweeten with a little honey, maple syrup or stevia, if necessary) | **Rice Salad with Dino Kale, Oranges & Walnuts and Spicy Black Bean Burgers**<br><br>1 cup Rice Salad with Dino Kale, Oranges & Walnuts, p. 110<br><br>1 Spicy Black Bean Burger, p. 121 |  |

| Dinner | Snacks | Evening Prep |
|---|---|---|
| **Don't Falafel the Wagon & Last-Minute Lemony Kale Salad**<br><br>1 serving of Don't Falafel the Wagon, p. 127<br><br>1 1/2 cups Last-Minute Lemony Kale Salad, p. 111<br><br>*set aside 1 serving of Falafel and 1 1/2 cups Kale Salad for tomorrow's lunch | Choose 2 snacks daily from the Snack List, p. 82. | Pre-cook the rice for tomorrow night's Rice Salad with Dino Kale, Oranges & Walnuts (p. 110) or if tomorrow night is busy, assemble salad completely and refrigerate overnight. |
| **Rice Salad with Dino Kale, Oranges & Walnuts and Spicy Black Bean Burgers**<br><br>1 cup Rice Salad with Dino Kale, Oranges & Walnuts, p. 110<br><br>1 Spicy Black Bean Burger, p. 121, topped with 1 tbsp Smoky Mayo, p. 144<br><br>1 cup steamed or raw broccoli<br><br>*set aside 1 Black Bean Burger and 1 cup Rice Salad with Dino Kale for tomorrow's lunch | Choose 2 snacks daily from the Snack List, p. 82. | Mama's Little Helper, p. 135, will cook in the crockpot while you are out tomorrow. Pre-browning your ground beef and chopping your veggies tonight will allow you to toss them in the crockpot quickly in the morning. |
| **Mama's Little Helper & Side Salad**<br><br>1 1/2 cups Mama's Little Helper, p. 135<br><br>with side salad: 1 cup greens, 1/2 to 1 cup chopped raw veggies of choice and 1 tbsp Beat the Band Balsamic, p. 142<br><br>*set aside 1 cup Mama's Little Helper for tomorrow's lunch | Choose 2 snacks daily from the Snack List, p. 82. | If tomorrow night is busy, consider pre-peeling and cubing your squash for the Oven-Baked Butternut Squash Risotto, p. 130. |

| | Breakfast | Lunch | |
|---|---|---|---|
| **4** | **Avocado Egg Toast**<br><br>1 serving Avocado Egg Toast, p. 94<br><br>coffee or tea (with cow's milk or unsweetened dairy alternative; sweeten with a little honey, maple syrup or stevia, if necessary) | **Mama's Little Helper & Side Salad**<br><br>1 cup leftover Mama's Little Helper, p. 135<br><br>with side salad: 1 cup greens, 1/2 to 1 cup chopped raw veggies of choice and 1 tbsp Beat the Band Balsamic, p. 142 | |
| **5** | **Mason Jar Mornings**<br><br>1 serving Mason Jar Mornings (p. 92); add fruit just before serving<br><br>coffee or tea (with cow's milk or unsweetened dairy alternative; sweeten with a little honey, maple syrup or stevia, if necessary) | **Oven-Baked Butternut Squash Risotto & Side Salad or Soup**<br><br>1 cup Oven-Baked Butternut Squash Risotto, p. 130<br><br>with side salad: 1 cup greens, 1/2 to 1 cup chopped raw veggies of choice and 1 tbsp Beat the Band Balsamic, p. 142<br><br>or 1 cup Lemon-Basil Tomato Soup, p. 98 | |
| **6** | **Rice Bowls with Fried Egg and Sweet & Smoky Sauce**<br><br>1 serving Rice Bowls with Fried Egg and Sweet & Smoky Sauce, p. 95<br><br>coffee or tea (with cow's milk or unsweetened dairy alternative; sweeten with a little honey, maple syrup or stevia, if necessary) | **The Big Salad**<br><br>2 cups salad greens; 1/2 cup chopped grilled chicken, fish, tofu or beans of choice; 1 cup chopped raw veggies; 1 tsp sunflower or pumpkin seeds; 2 tbsp Beat the Band Balsamic, p. 142<br><br>1 piece of fruit | |

| Dinner | Snacks | Evening Prep |
|---|---|---|
| **Oven-Baked Butternut Squash Risotto & Side Salad**<br><br>1 1/2 cups Oven-Baked Butternut Squash Risotto, p. 130<br><br>with side salad: 1 cup greens, 1/2 to 1 cup chopped raw veggies of choice and 1 tbsp Beat the Band Balsamic, p. 142<br><br>*set aside 1 cup Risotto for tomorrow's lunch | Choose 2 snacks daily from the Snack List, p. 82. | Assemble Mason Jar Mornings (p. 92) for tomorrow's breakfast and refrigerate overnight to allow it to soak<br><br>Consider pre-cooking brown rice for tomorrow night's dinner if you'll be short on time. |
| **Rice Bowls with Fried Egg and Sweet & Smoky Sauce**<br><br>1 serving Rice Bowls with Fried Egg and Sweet & Smoky Sauce, p. 95<br><br>1 fruit or 1 cup berries<br><br>*set aside 1/2 cup cooked rice and 2 tbsp sauce for tomorrow's breakfast | Choose 2 snacks daily from the Snack List, p. 82. | |
| **Stir It Up!**<br>1 serving of Stir It Up! with Nutty Lime or Simple Stir-fry Sauce, p. 139<br><br>served over 1/2 cup brown rice or quinoa<br><br>*set aside 1 serving of Stir It Up and 1/2 cup rice for tomorrow's lunch | Choose 2 snacks daily from the Snack List, p. 82. | |

|   | Breakfast | Lunch |   |
|---|-----------|-------|---|
| 7 | **Avocado Egg Toast**<br><br>1 serving Avocado Egg Toast, p. 94<br><br>coffee or tea (with cow's milk or unsweetened dairy alternative; sweeten with a little honey, maple syrup or stevia, if necessary) | **Stir It Up!**<br><br>1 serving of Stir It Up! with Nutty Lime or Simple Stir-fry Sauce, p. 139<br><br>served over 1/2 cup brown rice or quinoa |   |

## Cleanstart Snack List: Weeks 1–5

- banana with 1 tsp natural almond or peanut butter
- sliced apple with 1 tsp natural almond or peanut butter
- 1 cup raw veggies with 1/4 cup Easy Hummus, p. 145
- 1 brown rice cake with 1 tsp natural almond or peanut butter and 1 tbsp apple butter
- 1 piece of fruit or 1 cup berries with 12 almonds
- 1 hard-boiled egg with 1 cup cherry tomatoes, raw veggies or fruit
- 1 serving Pumpkin Pie Baked Oatmeal, p. 91
- 1 Roasted Red Pepper & Kale Egg Cup, p. 89 and 1/2 a banana
- 2 (small) Cocoa-Nut Lime Power Balls, p. 148
- 2 dried dates and 12 almonds
- 3 tbsp organic corn kernels popped in 2 tsp coconut oil (or air-popped)
- 1/2 cup plain greek yoghurt with 1 cup berries or 1/2 banana, 1 tbsp flax, chia, or chopped walnuts & 1 tsp maple syrup

| Dinner | Snacks | Evening Prep |
|--------|--------|--------------|
| **This Chalet Chicken, Nutty Napa Slaw & Sweet Potato Wedges**<br><br>3/4 cup This Chalet Chicken (without skin), p. 131<br><br>1 cup Nutty Napa Slaw, p. 107<br><br>1 cup Sweet Potato Wedges, p. 116<br><br>*consider roasting 2 chickens and slicing and freezing the second for future meals | Choose 2 snacks daily from the Snack List, p. 82. | |

# PART 3
# THE RECIPES

CF = CLEANSTART-FRIENDLY

DF = DAIRY-FREE

GF = GLUTEN-FREE

V = VEGETARIAN

VG = VEGAN

CFO = CLEANSTART-FRIENDLY OPTION

DFO = DAIRY-FREE OPTION

GFO = GLUTEN-FREE OPTION

VO = VEGETARIAN OPTION

VGO = VEGAN OPTION

# CHAPTER 13

## Breakfast

### Cinnamon Oats & Berries
*VG, DF, GF, CFO*

My most basic breakfast recipe — this might just become your busy morning go-to. The oats have lasting power when combined with healthy fat and fibre from the flax and fruit. For an even more convenient breakfast — when travelling, for example — pre-portion instant oats, flax, cinnamon and stevia in a heatproof container. In the morning, add your hot water and fruit and you're good to go.

1/4 cup plain instant, slow-cook, or steel-cut oats *
1 tbsp ground flax or chopped walnuts
1/4 tsp cinnamon
2 tbsp unsweetened applesauce
dash of vanilla extract
1/4 cup fresh or frozen berries, or a chopped or grated apple or pear
1/2 tsp maple syrup or stevia to taste**

To make: Cook oats in water according to package directions (cooking times will vary depending on the type of oats you prefer to use). Add flax or nuts, cinnamon, applesauce, vanilla, berries or other fruit and stir to combine.

Taste first, and if you need more sweetness, add 1/2 tsp of maple syrup (or a little stevia, if you're in the Cleanstart week).

*Serves 1.*

**\* to ensure recipe is gluten-free, use certified gluten-free oats**

**\*\*added sweetener is optional. If you need some during the Cleanstart week, use stevia only.**

## Eggs with Sautéed Greens & Avocado

*V, DF, GF, CF*

In the colder fall and winter months, I start most of my days with this simple, satisfying meal. The eggs are high in protein, the avocado provides a hit of healthy fat and you're guaranteed a couple of servings of veggies before you're even out the door. It takes just five minutes to make and dirties only one pan. Can't beat that!

1/2 tsp olive oil
1 egg
1/4 cup pure liquid egg whites
1 green onion, chopped (or 1 tbsp chopped onion or shallot)
1 1/2 cups washed baby spinach, kale or chard, coarsely chopped
1/2 cup chopped tomato or about 10 grape tomatoes, halved
1/8 of an avocado, peeled and sliced
sea salt & black pepper to taste

To make: Heat olive oil in medium-sized pan over medium heat. Add egg and egg whites to one side of pan. While the egg mixture is cooking, cook onion, spinach and tomato on the other side of the pan.

Once eggs are cooked, plate them and top with sautéed veggies, sliced avocado and salt and pepper to taste.

*Serves 1.*

## Anytime Tofu Scramble

*VG, DF ,G F, CF*

This is my homemade version of the yummy scrambled tofu I always order at my favourite brunch spot. Serve this with fruit and toast for a cheap and cheerful breakfast, lunch or dinner! Remember to always look for organic tofu to avoid genetically modified soy.

2 tsp coconut oil
1/2 cup finely chopped onion
2 to 3 green onions, finely chopped
1 to 2 cloves garlic, crushed
1 red bell pepper, finely chopped (or 1/2 cup jarred roasted red peppers, drained and finely chopped)
1 package (454 g) firm organic tofu
1/2 tsp ground cumin
1/2 tsp turmeric
1/4 tsp ground coriander
1/4 tsp dried thyme
1/8 tsp chili powder
1/8 tsp paprika
1/8 tsp salt
1/8 tsp black pepper

To make: Melt coconut oil in a large skillet and add onion, green onions, garlic and red pepper. Cook until softened, about 3 to 5 minutes.

Drain tofu of excess water and cut into slabs, then crumble tofu into the pan in bite-sized pieces.

Meanwhile, combine cumin, turmeric, coriander, thyme, chili powder, paprika, salt and pepper in a small dish.

Add spice mixture to tofu and mix well. Cook about 5 minutes more or until heated through.

*Serves 4 to 5.*

## Roasted Red Pepper & Kale Egg Cups

*V, DF, GF, CF*

Make this simple recipe in advance and freeze, then defrost and heat for a quick pop of protein in the morning, as a snack or with a salad for lunch.

2 tsp olive oil, divided
1/2 cup finely chopped roasted red pepper (if using jarred, drain first)
2 green onions, chopped
2 cups finely chopped curly kale
6 to 8 large whole leaves curly kale
10 eggs
1/4 cup almond, soy or cow's milk
1/2 cup nutritional yeast
1 garlic clove, crushed
1 tsp dried basil
1/2 tsp black pepper
1/4 tsp sea salt

To make: Grease 12 muffin tin cups *very* well with 1 tsp olive oil.

In a large saucepan, heat 1 tsp oil over medium heat. Add red pepper, green onions and chopped kale and cook about 5 minutes, until softened. Remove from heat and let cool slightly.

Meanwhile, in a large bowl, whisk eggs, then gently stir in milk, nutritional yeast, garlic, basil, pepper and salt. Stir the cooked veggies into the egg mixture.

In each greased muffin cup, overlap a couple of torn pieces of the whole kale leaves (discarding the centre stems) with the curly edge at the top, to cover the bottom and sides and form a "liner." Divide the egg mixture equally amongst the 12 kale-lined muffin cups, gently pouring about 1/3 cup in each.

Bake at 350°F for 22 to 25 minutes or until tops are no longer wet. Remove from oven and let cool for 5 minutes, then gently run knife around the edges and lift egg cups out and place on a rack to cool. The centres may deflate slightly, but don't panic, this is normal!

*Makes 12 egg cups.*

## Portobello Eggs Benny With Cashew Hollandaise

*V, DF, GF*

This lemony, cashew hollandaise is out of this world. You'd never know it was vegan. Make the sauce and spoon over eggs and sautéed veggies, or go big and assemble the full Eggs Benny. Don't forget to set your cashews out to soak at least 3 hours in advance (they can be left to soak in the fridge overnight if that's easier).

### Cashew Hollandaise

1/2 cup cashews
1/2 tsp grated lemon rind
2 tbsp lemon juice
1 tsp apple cider vinegar
1 tbsp chopped onion
1 tbsp nutritional yeast
1/8 tsp sea salt
1/8 tsp black pepper
1/8 tsp turmeric
pinch to 1/8 tsp cayenne (depending on how spicy you like it!)
1/3 cup water

### Portobello Eggs Benny (1 serving)

1 egg
1 portobello mushroom cap
olive oil
balsamic vinegar

To make: In a medium bowl, cover cashews in water and soak for at least 3 hours. Drain cashews.

In a food processor, combine soaked cashews, lemon rind and juice, vinegar, onion, nutritional yeast, salt, pepper, turmeric and cayenne and blend. Slowly add the water while blending, starting with 1/4 cup and adding more to thin to desired consistency.

For Portobello Eggs Benny, poach an egg for about 6 to 7 minutes or until cooked to desired consistency. In the meantime, brush a portobello cap with olive oil & balsamic oil and bake at 400°F for about 10 to 15 minutes. I lay my caps right on a cookie cooling rack and place that directly on the oven rack. You can also use an outdoor grill.

Layer cooked mushroom cap and poached egg and top with 1 1/2 tbsp Cashew Hollandaise. You can use half of a 100% whole grain English muffin or slice of Ezekiel sprouted grain toast as your base.

*Makes about 10 tbsp sauce, or 6 servings.*

## Pumpkin Pie Baked Oatmeal
*VG, DF, GF, CFO*

This is a simple, delicious make-ahead breakfast that can also be eaten cold for a quick, energy-rich snack. Warm it up in the morning and top with some sliced bananas, applesauce or Greek yoghurt. Drizzle it with a little maple syrup if you're feeling indulgent, but stick to stevia as a sweetener if you're following the Cleanstart program.

2 cups slow-cook rolled oats*
1/2 cup oat bran*
2 tsp pumpkin pie spice**
2 tsp aluminum-free baking powder
1/4 tsp sea salt
1 apple, cored and cut into 1/2-inch cubes (unpeeled if it's organic)
1/4 cup pumpkin seeds
1 1/2 cups unsweetened pumpkin purée
3 tbsp maple syrup (or 3/4 tsp powdered stevia***)
3/4 cup unsweetened almond (or cow's***) milk

**\*to ensure recipe is gluten-free, use certified gluten-free oats**

**\*\*If you don't have premixed pumpkin pie spice, you can make your own by combining 4 tbsp cinnamon, 4 tsp ground nutmeg, 4 tsp ground ginger and 3 tsp allspice. Store remainder in an airtight jar.**

**\*\*\* use stevia and almond milk if you are following Cleanstart**

To make: Lightly grease an 8- x 8-inch baking dish.

In a large bowl, combine oats, bran, pumpkin pie spice, baking powder, salt, apple and pumpkin seeds.

In a medium bowl, whisk together pumpkin purée, maple syrup (or stevia, if you're following Cleanstart) and milk.

Add wet to dry and stir to combine well. Pour mixture in baking dish, distributing evenly, and bake at 350°F for 30 to 35 minutes or until inserted toothpick comes out clean.

Enjoy warm or refrigerate for the next morning. This also freezes well, so I often pre-portion, then freeze.

*Serves 9.*

## Mason Jar Mornings

*VG, DF, GF*

Simplest breakfast for a busy parent? Mason jar oats. Assemble these the night before, let them sit in the fridge overnight and simply grab and go in the morning.

1/4 cup dry steel-cut oats* 1 tbsp shredded unsweetened coconut
2 tsp raw, shelled sunflower seeds
1 medjool date, finely chopped
1/2 tsp vanilla extract
1/3 cup unsweetened almond, soy or cow's milk
1/2 cup chopped fresh or defrosted frozen strawberries

**\* to ensure recipe is gluten-free, use certified gluten-free oats and oat bran**

To make: Combine oats, coconut, sunflower seeds, date, vanilla and milk in a Mason jar, stir well, then cover with lid and let sit in the fridge overnight. No need to cook, as the oats will soften on their own. In the morning, add strawberries and enjoy!

*Serves 1.*

## Zucchini Pie with Tarragon Asiago Rice Crust

*V, GF*

I love fresh tarragon with eggs, and I love quiche, but what I don't love is making pastry. This recipe is the perfect way to avoid pastry, impress a brunch or dinner crowd and use up your leftover rice. Rice is a great solution for a whole grain savoury pie crust if you're avoiding or just cutting back on gluten. Pre-cooked quinoa also works well in its place.

### Crust

1 1/2 cups pre-cooked, cooled brown rice (or quinoa)
1 tbsp chopped fresh tarragon
1/3 cup grated Asiago cheese
1 large egg white (or 3 tbsp liquid egg whites)
1/4 tsp sea salt
1/4 tsp black pepper

### Filling

6 eggs
1/2 cup unsweetened almond (or cow's) milk
1 tbsp Dijon mustard
1/2 tsp sea salt
1/2 tsp black pepper
1 small zucchini, unpeeled and grated
3 green onions, finely chopped
1 medium tomato or a few grape tomatoes, sliced
1/2 tsp (or more) chopped fresh tarragon, to garnish

To make: Combine the rice, tarragon, Asiago, egg white, salt and pepper together in a medium bowl until a sticky mixture forms. Press mixture into a greased pie plate to form a crust (no need to go more than 3/4 of the way up the side of the pan). The mixture will seem loose, but as it cooks it will set together. Bake the crust at 425°F for 12 minutes. Remove crust from oven to cool slightly.

Meanwhile, in a medium bowl, whisk eggs, milk, mustard, salt and pepper, then add zucchini and green onion. Pour mixture into crust and garnish with tomato and tarragon.

Bake at 425°F for 15 minutes, then reduce heat to 350°F and continue baking for 20 to 25 minutes, or until eggs are set and top is dry.

*Serves 6 as a main course.*

## Avocado Egg Toast

*V, DF*

There's something kind of decadent about slathering creamy avocado onto toast and topping it with a fried egg — comfort food at its best. You can keep it simple or take it up a notch with a crush of garlic, dash of hot sauce or pinch of crushed red pepper.

1 slice Ezekiel sprouted grain bread, toasted
1/4 of an avocado
squeeze of lemon or lime juice
sea salt to taste
1 egg
1/2 tsp olive oil
alfalfa sprouts, sliced tomato or arugula, to garnish (optional)

To make: In a small bowl, or right on the toast, mash together the avocado, lemon juice and salt (or experiment with a little kick in the form of garlic, hot sauce or crushed red pepper).

Fry your egg in a non-stick pan or in the oil and lay it on top of the avocado.

To garnish, add as desired: sprouts, sliced tomato or arugula — all lovely additions to this quick breakfast.

*Serves 1.*

## PB & J Breakfast Smoothie

*VG, DF, GF*

Who doesn't love PB & J? Try this quick, healthy smoothie for a grab-and-go breakfast. You can add some clean protein powder if you're using it as a recovery meal after a hardcore, sweaty workout.

1 cup fresh or frozen strawberries
2 tsp natural peanut or almond butter
1/2 cup unsweetened almond (or cow's) milk
1/2 cup packed fresh baby spinach
1/2 fresh or frozen banana
1/2 cup water

To make: Blend berries, peanut butter, almond milk, spinach, banana and water. Serve and enjoy!

*Serves 1.*

## Rice Bowls with Fried Egg and Sweet & Smoky Sauce

*V, DF, GF*

These bowls make a perfect weekend brunch or lunch, and they just so happen to be gluten- and dairy-free! A fried egg and crispy sesame kale up the ante, the sauce whips up in 3 minutes in a food processor or good blender and if you have leftover cooked rice you can throw the rest together in about 5 minutes.

### Sweet & Smoky Sauce

1 green onion
2 tbsp tahini
2 tbsp water
2 tsp lemon or lime juice
1 tsp low-sodium soy sauce or tamari
1 tsp apple cider vinegar
1 tsp maple syrup
1 garlic clove
1/2 tsp toasted sesame oil (or regular sesame oil, if you can't find toasted)
1/4 tsp chili powder
1/4 tsp smoked paprika*

### Rice Bowl (makes 4 bowls)

2 tsp toasted (or regular) sesame oil
4 eggs
4 cups chopped kale
2 cups thinly sliced, chopped cabbage
2 cups cooked brown rice
sesame seeds, to garnish (optional)

**\*if you don't like the "smoky" flavour this spice imparts, use regular paprika instead**

To make: To make the sauce, blend the onion, tahini, water, lemon juice, soy sauce, vinegar, maple syrup, garlic, sesame oil, chili powder and paprika in a food processor until smooth.

To make the Rice Bowl, heat the sesame oil in a pan over medium heat. Add an egg to one side of the pan and add 1 cup kale and 1/4 cup cabbage to the other. While the egg cooks to desired consistency, turn the kale regularly to allow it to "crisp" a bit (it's almost like toasting it). Place 1/2 cup rice in bowl, top with kale and cabbage and 1 fried egg. Garnish bowl with 2 tbsp of the prepared sauce and a sprinkle of sesame seeds, if using. Repeat for other bowls, or cook all the eggs and veggies at once in a very large pan.

*Serves 4.*

## Southwestern Black Bean Frittata

*V, DF, DFO, CFO*

Quick and delicious, this dairy-free, high-protein dish works for breakfast, lunch or dinner. Serve with a side of greens and a Sweet P Biscuit (p. 146) for a gourmet meal. It's an ultra-flexible recipe: you can substitute any bean for the black beans, arugula or baby kale for the spinach and basil for the cilantro.

1 tbsp olive oil
1 medium onion, diced
1 1/2 cups diced peeled butternut squash or pumpkin
8 eggs
1 can (14 oz/398 mL) black beans, rinsed (or 1 1/2 cups cooked)
1 cup spinach, packed then finely chopped
1/4 cup packed fresh parsley, finely chopped
1/4 cup packed fresh cilantro, finely chopped
1/4 tsp sea salt
1/4 tsp black pepper
1/8 tsp nutmeg
1/4 cups grated Asiago or Parmesan cheese (*optional)

**\*to keep this dairy-free and Cleanstart-friendly, omit cheese**

To make: In a cast iron pan, heat olive oil over medium heat. Add onion and squash and cook for 10 minutes, covering halfway and stirring occasionally, until squash is a bit tender. Remove from heat and spread squash mixture evenly to cover bottom of pan.

Whisk eggs in a large bowl. Stir in beans, spinach, parsley, cilantro, salt, pepper and nutmeg. Pour into cast iron pan over onion and squash mixture. Sprinkle grated cheese over the top, if using.

Place pan in oven and bake at 350°F for about 30 minutes, or until top is set and no longer looks wet.

*Serves 8.*

# The Breakfast Salad

*V, DF, GF, CF*

What's the best way to start the day? With a salad, of course! You'll feel great leaving the house with a few servings of veggies already under your belt, trust me! This is my go-to warmer weather breakfast — I love to throw in fresh herbs for a hit of summer freshness when I have them on hand.

1 egg
1/4 cup pure liquid egg whites
2 cups salad greens (try spinach or arugula)
1/2 cup chopped tomato or sliced grape tomatoes
1/8 avocado, sliced
1 1/2 tbsp Green Goddess Dressing, p. 143
(or any other dressing recipe found in Salad Dressings & Sauces)

To make: In a non-stick or lightly oiled pan, scramble or fry the egg and egg whites to your preferred consistency. Place the salad greens in a large bowl, top with tomato and avocado, then with cooked egg and drizzle with dressing.

# CHAPTER 14

## Lunch

### Lemon-Basil Tomato Soup

*VG, DF, GF, CF*

This lunch box–friendly soup is so easy and so good — my kids and husband love it.

1 tbsp olive oil
3 small shallots, chopped
1 garlic clove, crushed
1 can or jar (28 oz/796 mL) no-salt-added whole tomatoes
2 cups low-sodium vegetable broth
1/3 cup fresh basil
1 tbsp grated lemon rind (rind of about 1 lemon)
1/4 cup nutritional yeast
1 tsp sea salt (or more to taste)
1/2 tsp black pepper
1 1/2 cups cooked white beans (or 1 can [14 oz/398 mL], well rinsed)

To make: In a soup pot, heat oil over medium heat. Add shallots and garlic, and cook for a few minutes until shallots are translucent.

Stir in tomatoes, broth, basil, lemon rind, nutritional yeast, salt, pepper and beans. Bring to a boil, then remove pot from heat and let cool slightly.

Blend with an immersion blender or in batches in a stand blender, adding more salt to taste if necessary.

*Makes 8 cups.*

## Smoky Broccoli Soup

*VG, DF, GF, CF*

This mouthwatering soup has a complex flavour. It's creamy, yet dairy-free, and cheesy, but cheese-free. Trust me, you really can make that magic happen with the right blend of ingredients!

1 tbsp coconut oil
3 shallots, or 1 yellow onion, chopped
1 garlic clove, crushed
1 medium potato, peeled and cubed
1 carrot, peeled and sliced
1 rib celery, sliced
2 tbsp arrowroot powder
1 1/2 cups unsweetened almond milk, divided*
2 cups low-sodium vegetable broth
1/3 cup nutritional yeast
1/4 tsp nutmeg
1/2 tsp smoked paprika**
1/2 tsp salt
1/2 tsp black pepper
1 large or 2 small heads broccoli, including stalk, chopped

**\*you can use cow's milk if you are not avoiding dairy or following Cleanstart**

**\*\*if you don't like the "smoky" flavour this spice imparts, use regular paprika instead**

To make: Melt oil in a soup pot over medium heat. Add shallots and garlic and cook for a few minutes until softened. Add potato, carrot and celery and stir, cooking another 5 minutes or so.

In a small bowl, whisk arrowroot into 1/2 cup of the almond milk. Add this mixture to the veggies in the soup pot and stir well. Add the remaining 1 cup of almond milk, broth, nutritional yeast, nutmeg, paprika, salt and pepper. Bring to a low boil, then reduce to a simmer, stirring occasionally so it doesn't stick to the bottom, and cook for 10 minutes or until potatoes are just tender. Add broccoli and simmer for another 15 to 20 minutes or until broccoli is soft. Remove from heat and blend to a creamy consistency with an immersion or stand blender.

*Makes about 7 cups.*

## Beta Butternut Soup

*VG, DF, GF, CF*

Get your daily dose of beta carotene and vitamin C in this delicious, warming mug of comfort. Roast your squash and sweet potato in advance for a quicker weeknight meal.

1 medium butternut squash
1 medium sweet potato
1 tbsp coconut oil
1/2 cup chopped onion or shallot
3 cloves garlic, crushed
2 carrots, peeled and thinly sliced
2 ribs celery, sliced
2 cups low-sodium vegetable broth
1/2 cup unsweetened applesauce
4 cups water
1/2 tsp black pepper
3/4 tsp dried thyme
1 tbsp fresh rosemary (or 1 tsp dried)
3/4 tsp nutmeg
1 to 1 1/2 tsp salt (taste after 1 tsp, and add more if you need)

To make: Cut squash in half, scoop out seeds and lay halves skin-side up on a lightly sprayed baking pan. Place the sweet potato on the same pan, unpeeled, with a few holes poked into its skin. Roast squash and sweet potato at 400°F for about 45 minutes, or until tender. Remove from oven and let cool. Peel and chop both into chunks.

In a soup pot, melt oil over medium heat, then cook onions, garlic, carrots and celery until slightly softened.

Add the broth, applesauce, water, roasted squash and sweet potato, pepper, thyme, rosemary, nutmeg and 1 tsp of salt. Bring to a boil and then reduce to a simmer, cooking for about 20 minutes or until the carrots and celery are quite soft. Blend the mixture with an immersion or stand blender, tasting after blending and adding more salt if necessary.

*Makes about 12 cups.*

## Thai This Soup

*VG, GF, DF, CF*

This deliciously warming soup was inspired by a viciously cold snap, a jar of red curry paste and a bunch of fresh cilantro. Thai This Soup, you won't regret it!

2 tsp coconut oil
1 medium yellow onion, chopped
2 to 3 garlic cloves, crushed
1 tbsp + 1 tsp red curry or harissa paste
1 tsp ground cumin
1 tsp ground coriander
1 tsp dried basil
4 cups low-sodium vegetable broth
2 cups water
1 1/4 cups dry yellow split peas, rinsed
1 medium carrot, peeled and finely grated
1 can (28 oz/796 mL) whole tomatoes
1 tbsp grated fresh ginger (or 1 tsp dried)
1 can (400 mL) light coconut milk
1/3 cup packed fresh cilantro, chopped
2 tsp grated lime rind (rind of 1 lime)
1 tbsp lime juice (about 1 lime)
3/4 to 1 tsp sea salt, to taste
chopped green onions, to garnish (optional)

To make: Melt coconut oil in a large soup pot. Add onion and garlic and cook until onion is softened, then stir in curry paste, cumin, coriander and basil. Add broth, water, split peas, carrot, tomatoes, and ginger and bring to a boil. Reduce to a medium simmer and cover. Let cook about 50 to 60 minutes, or until split peas are tender, stirring occasionally.

Add coconut milk, cilantro, lime rind and juice and heat through. Remove from heat. Purée with immersion blender or in stand blender and add salt as needed to taste. Serve alone or over rice garnished with chopped green onions. If you refrigerate or freeze after making, you may want to add a little stock or water when you reheat to thin it back out.

*Makes about 12 cups.*

## Sopa Negro

*DFO, GF, CFO*

Before we had children, we took a (very) low-budget trip to Costa Rica, where we backpacked, took a rickety bus through the mountains, rode horses with a friendly Rastafarian guide named Mr. Joseph to a hidden waterfall and drank cold beer on the beach. We also ate a whole lot of "Sopa Negro," or Black Bean Soup. It was so divine I just had to recreate that lovely Latin flavour.

1 tbsp olive oil
1 yellow onion, chopped
4 garlic cloves, chopped
1 tbsp chili powder
2 tsp ground cumin
1/2 tsp sea salt
1/4 tsp black pepper
1/4 tsp smoked paprika*
2 cans (each 14 oz/398 mL) black beans, rinsed (or 3 cups cooked from dry)
1 can (28 oz/796 mL) diced tomatoes
2 cups low-sodium vegetable broth
2 tsp grated lime rind
1 tbsp lime juice
1/2 cup packed cilantro, chopped
plain Greek yoghurt, to garnish**
avocado, to garnish

**\*if you don't like the "smoky" flavour this spice imparts, use regular paprika instead**

**\*\*omit to keep this dairy-free and Cleanstart-friendly**

To make: In a large soup pot, heat olive oil over medium heat. Cook onion and garlic until softened, then stir in chili powder, cumin, salt, pepper and paprika. Add beans, diced tomatoes and broth and bring to a boil. Reduce heat to a simmer and stir in lime rind and juice and chopped cilantro. Let simmer about 10 minutes, then remove from heat and purée with an immersion blender or in batches in a stand blender until almost smooth. If you like a chunkier soup, reserve 2 cups of the soup before blending, then add back to the pot once you've blended the rest.

Serve topped with a spoonful of plain Greek yoghurt and chopped avocado.

*Makes 6 cups.*

## Syrian Lentil Soup

*VG, DF, GF, CF*

When I asked the owner of my family's favourite Syrian restaurant what went into his popular lentil soup, he said: "No stock — just water, red lentils and spice." Determined to replicate it, I came up with this version. Quick and budget-friendly, this lemony lentil soup is now one of our favourites.

2 tsp coconut oil
1 medium onion, chopped
2 garlic cloves, crushed
2 cups red lentils, picked over and rinsed
8 cups water
2 tbsp grated lemon rind (rind of 2 lemons)
1/4 cup lemon juice (about 2 lemons)
2 1/2 tsp sea salt
2 tsp ground cumin
1/2 tsp ground coriander
1/2 tsp black pepper

To make: In a large soup pot, melt coconut oil over medium heat, then add onions and garlic and cook a few minutes until onion is softened. Add lentils, water, lemon rind and juice, salt, cumin, coriander and pepper and bring to a boil. Reduce heat to a simmer and cover. Cook for 18 minutes or until lentils are softened.

*Makes about 10 cups.*

## Mexican Chicken Soup

*DF, GFO, CFO*

Lime, fresh cilantro, allspice and just a hint of chili make for a delicious, Latin-inspired twist on chicken soup.

1 tbsp olive or coconut oil
1 lb (454 g) boneless chicken breasts (about 2 medium breasts), cut into 1-inch cubes
1 cup chopped onion
2 garlic cloves, crushed
8 cups low-sodium chicken broth
4 medium tomatoes, diced
1/2 cup packed fresh cilantro, chopped
1 tsp dried oregano
1/2 tsp allspice
1/4 tsp black pepper
1/8 tsp crushed red pepper
2 cups finely chopped fresh spinach
1 tbsp grated lime rind (about 1 lime)
2 tbsp lime juice 1/2 to 1 tsp sea salt
4 cups pre-cooked whole grain or gluten-free penne or fusilli (optional*)

**\*to keep this recipe gluten-free, use gluten-free pasta; to keep it Cleanstart-friendly, omit pasta and substitute 2 cup pre-cooked brown rice**

To make: In a large soup pot, melt oil over medium, then add chopped chicken, onions, and garlic and cook, stirring, until chicken is cooked through.

Add broth, tomatoes, cilantro, oregano, allspice, pepper and crushed red pepper. Bring to a boil, then reduce heat and simmer for 5 minutes. Add the spinach, lime rind and juice and let simmer about 5 minutes longer. Add sea salt to taste. If using noodles, add them after salting the soup and allow noodles to heat through.

*Makes about 12 cups without noodles or 15 cups with noodles.*

## Cancun Quinoa

*VG, DF, GF, CF*

This quick, summery salad stores for a few days in the fridge and serves up lots of protein and fibre in a zesty Mexican dressing. If you've pre-cooked your quinoa, it whips up in five minutes and makes a great lunch over greens or an easy side with dinner.

2 cups cooked quinoa
2 tomatoes, coarsely chopped
1 can (14 oz/398 mL) black beans, rinsed well (or 1 1/2 cups cooked)
1/2 cup chopped red onion
1 cup organic fresh or frozen corn kernels, cooked and cooled
2 tsp flax oil
4 tbsp lime juice
1 tbsp chopped fresh cilantro (or 1 tsp dried)
1/2 tsp chili powder
1/2 tsp ground cumin
1/8 tsp sea salt
1 avocado, peeled, pitted and sliced, to garnish

To make: In a large bowl, combine quinoa, tomatoes, beans, onion and corn.

In a small bowl or glass measuring cup, whisk together oil, lime juice, cilantro, chili powder, cumin and salt.

Combine dressing with salad and mix well. Top each serving with a couple of slices of avocado.

*Makes about 5 1/2 cups.*

## Chickpea Tabbouleh

*VG, DF, GF, CF*

This is a delicious, nutritious, high-protein lunch that stores and travels easily. Cook your quinoa in advance on the stove or in a rice cooker to save time. Don't skimp on the fresh herbs — they really make this salad!

1 cup quinoa, well rinsed and drained
1 1/4 cups water
1 large cucumber, peeled, quartered and sliced
20 cherry tomatoes, quartered (or 2 medium tomatoes, coarsely chopped)
1 can (14 oz/398 mL) chickpeas, rinsed (or 1 1/2 cups cooked chickpeas)
1/3 cup minced red onion
1/2 cup chopped fresh mint
1/2 cup chopped fresh parsley
1/3 cup lemon juice
3 tbsp olive oil
2 tbsp apple cider vinegar
2 garlic cloves, crushed
1/4 tsp black pepper
1/4 tsp sea salt

To make: Combine quinoa and water in medium pot and bring to a boil. Reduce to medium-low heat, cover and cook for 15 to 20 minutes or until quinoa is tender. Transfer to bowl and let cool.

Meanwhile, combine cucumber, tomatoes, chickpeas, onion, mint and parsley in salad bowl.

In separate bowl or glass measuring cup, whisk together lemon juice, olive oil, vinegar, garlic, pepper and salt.

Add cooled quinoa to vegetable mixture, then pour dressing over top and toss well. Store in an airtight container in the fridge — the longer it sits, the better it tastes!

*Makes about 6 cups.*

## Nutty Napa Slaw

*VG, DF, GF, CFO*

This is a crowd-pleasing coleslaw that makes a lovely side with grilled meat or fish, or a light lunch with some chickpeas or cooked chicken tossed in for added protein.

8 cups shredded napa cabbage (about 1 small to medium cabbage)
1 cup shredded purple cabbage (about 1/2 small cabbage)
2 cups grated carrots (about 4 small carrots)
1/4 cup packed chopped fresh cilantro, divided
1/4 cup chopped peanuts or cashews, divided*
2 tbsp natural peanut butter or almond butter*
1 tbsp low-sodium soy sauce or tamari
2 tbsp white wine vinegar or apple cider vinegar*
1 large garlic clove, crushed
1 tsp grated fresh ginger
3 tbsp water
1/8 to 1/4 tsp crushed red pepper, to taste

**\*use cashews, almond butter and apple cider vinegar during Cleanstart week**

To make: In a large bowl, combine cabbage, carrots and 3 tbsp each of the cilantro and nuts, reserving 1 tbsp cilantro for dressing and 1 tbsp nuts for garnish.

Combine reserved 1 tbsp cilantro, peanut butter, soy sauce, vinegar, garlic, ginger, water and crushed red pepper (to taste, start with 1/8 tsp) in food processor and blend until smooth.

Toss dressing well with salad and top with reserved nuts.

*Makes 10 cups.*

## Sunshine Slaw

*V, DF, GF*

Sometimes you just need to make your own summer, especially when you live through a cold Canadian winter every year. This easy tropical slaw does the trick and makes a lovely side for just about any main dish.

4 cups grated or finely chopped cabbage, any type
1 large carrot, peeled and grated
1 apple, diced
1 orange, peeled, segmented and chopped
1/4 cup raisins
2 tbsp unsweetened finely shredded coconut
1/4 cup orange juice (fresh-squeezed is best!)
1 tbsp olive oil
1 tbsp white wine vinegar
1 tsp honey
1/4 tsp black pepper
1/8 tsp sea salt

To make: In a large bowl, combine cabbage, carrot, apple, orange, raisins and coconut. In a separate bowl or glass measuring cup, whisk together orange juice, oil, vinegar, honey, pepper and salt, then pour over slaw and toss well. Refrigerate for a few hours to amplify the sunny flavour.

*Makes about 7 cups.*

## Thai Rice Noodle Salad
*VGO, DF, GF*

This Asian-inspired, flavour-packed noodle salad will get you out of that lunch rut, pronto.

1 block (454 g) of extra-firm tofu*, 1 boneless chicken breast or 2 cups peeled shrimp
1 tsp coconut oil
1/2 lb rice noodles (half a 454 g package)
1 cup frozen, unshelled edamame, defrosted
1 carrot, cut into 2-inch-long thin matchsticks
3 green onions, sliced
1/4 cup packed fresh cilantro, chopped
2 tbsp natural peanut butter
2 tbsp apple cider vinegar
1/8 tsp crushed red pepper
2 tbsp low-sodium soy sauce or tamari
2 tsp tahini
2 tbsp water
1 garlic clove, crushed
2 tsp grated fresh ginger (or 3/4 tsp dried)
1 tbsp lime juice (about 1 lime)
2 tbsp chopped cashews or peanuts (optional)

**\*to keep this recipe vegan, use tofu**

To make: Cut tofu or chicken into 1/2-inch cubes. Cook either tofu, chicken or shrimp in 1 tsp coconut oil over medium heat until tofu is browned or the chicken or shrimp is cooked through. Remove from heat and set aside.

Fill a large kettle with water and boil. Place the rice noodles, edamame and carrots in a large bowl and cover completely with boiling water, using tongs to gently separate the noodles. Let sit until noodles are tender, about 5 to 10 minutes, depending on type of noodles you are using. Drain noodles once softened and toss in a bowl with tofu or chicken, green onions and cilantro.

Meanwhile, whisk together peanut butter, vinegar, crushed red pepper, soy sauce, tahini, water, garlic, ginger and lime juice.

Pour dressing over salad and mix well to coat evenly. Top with cashews for a little va-va-voom. Serve hot or cold.

*Makes about 8 cups.*

## Rice Salad with Dino Kale, Oranges & Walnuts

*VG, DF, GF*

This is an absolutely delicious recipe I've been tweaking for years. The final version is a whole grain, zesty, sweet dish packed with healthy omega-3s that makes a great side at dinnertime or a really satisfying lunch. It's all in the dressing, as you'll see!

4 cups cooked brown rice
2 cups finely chopped dinosaur kale (also known as lacinato or Tuscan kale), stems removed
1 orange, peeled, segmented, deseeded and chopped into small pieces
1/4 cup very finely chopped shallot or onion (I use a small food processor)
1/2 cup chopped walnuts
2 tbsp lime juice
2 tbsp flax or olive oil
1 tbsp balsamic vinegar
1 tbsp apple cider vinegar
1 tbsp maple syrup
2 tsp low-sodium soy sauce or tamari
1/8 tsp salt
1/8 tsp black pepper

To make: Combine rice, kale, orange pieces, shallot and walnuts in a large bowl.

In a measuring cup whisk together lime juice, oil, balsamic, apple cider vinegar, maple syrup, soy sauce, salt and pepper, then pour over rice mixture and stir to combine thoroughly.

You can eat this right away, but I prefer to let it sit in the fridge overnight to combine the flavours and soften the kale. Best served at room temperature.

*Makes about 8 cups.*

## Last-Minute Lemony Kale Salad

*V, GF*

You can assemble this in 5 minutes, give it another 5 minutes of massaging love (not kidding!) and presto — one tasty Lemony Kale Salad!

1 bunch kale, any type, washed, ribs removed, torn or sliced into ribbons
1/4 cup lemon juice (juice of about 1 lemon)
1/4 cup fresh finely grated Parmesan or Asiago cheese
1 garlic clove, crushed
1/4 tsp sea salt
1/8 tsp black pepper
3 tbsp olive oil

To make: Wash kale, remove ribs and tear or slice into ribbons. Place in a large bowl.

In a small bowl, combine lemon juice, cheese, garlic, salt and pepper in a bowl and whisk gently. Slowly add the olive oil, whisking to combine.

Pour dressing over the kale until completely coated (you may not need all of it), then massage the dressed kale with your hands for about 3 to 5 minutes, gently squeezing the leaves until they soften.

Serve with a little extra grated cheese on top.

You can dress this salad up with whole grain croutons or toasted nuts, but we love to keep it simple.

*Makes about 8 cups.*

## Smashed Chickpea Salad

*V, GF*

This is a truly addictive chickpea-based sandwich stuffer! Wrap it up with some spinach and sliced tomato in a whole grain pita or tortilla, or even in large lettuce leaves, for a gluten-free lunch.

1 can (14 oz/398 mL) chickpeas, rinsed and drained (or 1 1/2 cups cooked)
1/2 cup finely diced red onion
1/2 cup finely diced celery (about 1 medium rib)
1/2 cup shredded carrot (about 1 small carrot)
1/4 cup plain Greek yoghurt
2 tbsp tahini
1 tbsp Dijon mustard
2 tsp apple cider vinegar
1 tsp ground cumin
1/2 tsp smoked paprika*
1/4 tsp sea salt
1/4 tsp black pepper

**\*if you don't like the "smoky" flavour this spice imparts, use regular paprika instead**

To make: Pulse chickpeas in a food processor, or mash in a bowl with a fork or potato masher, until they've lost their shape. In a medium bowl, combine the onion, celery and carrot with the mashed chickpeas.

In a glass measuring cup or medium bowl, whisk together yoghurt, tahini, Dijon, vinegar, cumin, paprika, salt and pepper.

Add dressing to chickpea mixture and stir until well combined.

*Makes about 2 1/2 cups and serves 4 to 6.*

## Dillicious French Lentil Salad

*V, DFO, GF*

The distinctive peppery flavour of French lentils combined with fresh dill and creamy goat cheese make this salad dinner-party worthy. It will keep in your fridge for several days and travels well, so you can take leftovers for a lovely weekday lunch.

3 cups water
1 cup dried De Puy (French) lentils, picked over and rinsed
1 medium cucumber, diced
1 large or 2 small tomatoes, chopped
1/3 cup finely diced red onion
1/3 cup finely diced celery
1/3 cup packed chopped fresh parsley
1 tbsp chopped fresh dill
2 tbsp goat cheese (optional*)
2 tbsp + 1 tsp olive oil
2 tbsp red wine vinegar
2 tsp Dijon mustard
1 tsp honey
1/8 tsp sea salt

**\*to keep this recipe dairy-free, omit the cheese**

To make: Bring the water to a boil, add lentils, then cover and reduce heat, cooking for about 20 minutes or until lentils are tender. Remove from heat and drain.

In a large bowl, combine cooked lentils, cucumber, tomatoes, onion, celery, parsley, dill and goat cheese.

In a small bowl, whisk together oil, vinegar, mustard, honey and salt.

Pour dressing over salad and toss to combine well. Serve warm or cold.

*Serves 5 as a main course or 10 as a side dish.*

## Zesty Kale Caesar Salad

*V, DFO, VGO, GF, CFO*

This is the holy kitchen trifecta, as far as I'm concerned: simple, delicious and nutritious. If you're feeling all gourmet about it, top with some homemade croutons and even a little crumbled nitrate-free natural bacon.

1 large bunch curly kale
3 tbsp tahini
2 tsp grated lemon rind
3 tbsp lemon juice (about 1 lemon)
1/4 cup water
2 tbsp nutritional yeast
2 garlic cloves, crushed*
1 tsp Dijon mustard
1 tsp apple cider vinegar
1/2 tsp low-sodium soy sauce or tamari
1/8 tsp sea salt
1/8 tsp black pepper
2 tbsp grated Asiago or Parmesan cheese (optional**)
2 tbsp chopped toasted walnuts (optional)

**\*use more if you like your Caesar quite garlicky**

**\*\* to keep this recipe dairy-free, vegan and Cleanstart-friendly, omit the cheese**

To make: Clean kale, remove and discard stems and any large veins, and tear leaves into pieces. Place in salad bowl.

In a food processor or blender, combine tahini, lemon rind and juice, water, nutritional yeast, garlic, mustard, vinegar, soy sauce, salt and pepper and blend until smooth.

In a large salad bowl, combine kale with dressing and massage gently with your hands for 3 to 5 minutes, or until kale is softened and leaves are no longer tough.

Top with cheese and walnuts, if using, and serve.

*Serves 8 as a side salad. Makes about 1/2 cup dressing.*

## Warm Gribiche Salad

*V, DF, GFO*

Gribiche is a traditional mayo-style French dressing with a unique flavour, and my take on it, paired with roasted veggies and pasta, is now one of my most popular recipes. Don't forget to hard boil an egg and pre-cook your pasta before you get started. Prepare to be amazed!

1 1/2 lb baby potatoes (or 4 cups larger potatoes cubed to 1 inch)

2 tsp melted coconut oil

1 large head broccoli, cut into florets (about 6 cups florets)

16 oz (about 2 cups) cherry tomatoes

1 hard-boiled egg

1 tbsp tahini

1 tbsp capers (or 2 tbsp chopped dill pickle)

2 tsp red wine vinegar

1 tsp Dijon mustard

1 tbsp grated lemon rind (rind of 1 lemon)

3 tbsp lemon juice (about 1 lemon)

1/2 tsp sea salt

1/4 tsp black pepper

1 tbsp chopped onion or shallot

1 1/2 tbsp fresh tarragon

1 tbsp chives

2 tbsp chopped fresh parsley

1/4 cup olive oil

3 1/2 cups cooked whole grain penne or rotini pasta* (about 2 cups uncooked)

**\*to keep this recipe gluten-free, use gluten-free pasta**

To make: In a large bowl, toss potatoes with coconut oil and a pinch of sea salt. Spread the potatoes on a baking sheet, and roast at 400°F for 20 minutes. Remove pan from oven and add broccoli and tomatoes and carefully toss with the potato. Put the pan back in the oven for another 15 minutes or until potatoes are golden and tender.*

In a food processor, blend egg, tahini, capers, vinegar, mustard, lemon rind and juice, salt, pepper, onion, tarragon, chives and parsley until combined. While blending, slowly add olive oil to form a smooth dressing.

Transfer the veggies to a large bowl and toss with the pasta and dressing. Serve warm.

*Makes 11 to 12 cups. Dressing ingredients make 1 cup dressing.*

**\*Alternate cooking method: Cook potatoes in a grill basket on the barbecue, then add the other veggies and cook until they are all tender. Transfer to a large bowl and toss with dressing.**

# Oven-Roasted Veggies

*VG, DF, GF, CFO*

This recipe is a great way to clean out your pantry or fridge. I tend to use whatever veggies I have on hand, so it's usually a bit of a random mixture. You can use just about any vegetable in this recipe and it will taste amazing, so use your imagination! (Just aim for a total of about 8 cups of chopped vegetables.)

Here's a basic recipe to get you started:

1 tbsp coconut oil
2 cups peeled, cubed (into 1-inch pieces) yam or sweet potato
2 cups peeled, cubed (into 1-inch pieces) potato
1 cup peeled, cubed (into 1-inch pieces) carrot
2 cups quartered beets
2 cups brussels sprouts, washed, stems trimmed (slice very large sprouts lengthwise)
8 to 10 garlic cloves, peeled and cut lengthwise
1 onion, peeled and coarsely chopped
coarse sea salt and black pepper to taste
fresh or dried rosemary (totally optional)
2 tbsp balsamic vinegar (also optional*)

**\*to keep this recipe Cleanstart-friendly, omit the balsamic vinegar**

To make: Melt oil on stove or in the microwave. Add your prepped veggies to a roasting pan or an 11- x 9-inch baking dish and toss with oil to lightly coat. Sprinkle mixture with sea salt, pepper and a dash of rosemary, if using. Roast at 425°F for about 35 to 45 minutes, until veggies are tender, stirring occasionally.

Remove from oven and toss with the balsamic, if using, and more salt, if needed, to taste.

*Makes 7 cups.*

## Sweet Potato Wedges

*VG, DF, GF, CF*

The little black dress of side dishes, this basic, reliable recipe totally hits the spot and pairs well with any main dish, making it a meal-planning staple. Dress it up or dress it down.

2 medium sweet potatoes, peeled
1 tbsp olive oil
1/2 tsp paprika
a couple of pinches of sea salt

To make: Slice sweet potatoes to 1/2-inch thick rounds then slice into half-moons.

Combine the sweet potatoes, oil, paprika and salt in a bowl and toss to coat.

Spread potatoes on a baking sheet, taking care to keep the wedges from touching (this helps them crisp up) and roast at 400°F for 35 to 45 minutes, turning once or twice. Keep your eye on them to ensure they don't burn.

*Serves 4.*

# CHAPTER 15

## Dinner

## Salsa Burgers

*GF*

For a mouth-watering, zesty twist on a plain old burger, give these Salsa Burgers a try. You can use ground turkey, chicken, beef or pork and freeze leftover cooked patties.

2 lb (907 g) ground turkey, pork, chicken or beef
2/3 cup finely diced tomato
1/2 cup chopped red onion
1/2 cup fresh cilantro, packed, then finely chopped
2 garlic cloves, crushed
1 tsp smoked paprika*
1/8 tsp sea salt
1/8 tsp black pepper
1/2 cup grated Asiago, Parmesan or white cheddar cheese (optional)

**\*if you don't like the "smoky" flavour this spice imparts, use regular paprika instead**

To make: Combine turkey, tomato, onion, cilantro, garlic, paprika, salt, pepper and cheese, if using, in a large bowl and gently mix with your hands until just combined. Form into 8 patties.

If your grill is sticky, oil the grill or brush each patty with a little olive oil before placing on the grill.

Grill over medium-high heat for 6 to 8 minutes and then turn patties and grill for another 6 to 8 minutes, or until they are cooked through.

*Makes 8 patties.*

## Buddha Burgers

*V, DF, GF, CF*

The sauce from my popular Karmic Buddha Bowls (p. 122) inspired these uniquely seasoned veggie burgers. The beets' rich, earthy, almost "meaty" taste, combined with the umami flavourings, make these irresistibly good.

1 cup slow-cook rolled oats*

1/2 cup raw almonds

2 to 3 tbsp olive oil, divided

1 leek, white and light green part only, finely chopped

3 green onions, white and green parts, chopped

3 cloves garlic, crushed

3 medium beets, peeled and grated

2 tbsp apple cider vinegar

2 cups cooked green lentils (canned, or freshly cooked from about 3/4 cup dried)

3 eggs

1/4 cup low-sodium soy sauce or tamari

3 tbsp tahini

2 cups cooked quinoa (cooked from about 1 cup dry)

1/2 cup nutritional yeast

**\* to ensure recipe is gluten-free, use certified gluten-free oats**

To make: Grind oats to a flour in food processor, transfer to a bowl and set aside. Grind almonds to a raw meal, transfer to a bowl and set aside.

In a large pan, heat 1 tbsp of olive oil over medium heat. Add leek, onions and garlic and cook until softened, just a few minutes. Add beets and apple cider vinegar, and cook another few minutes until beets are softened. Remove from heat.

In food processor, pulse lentils, eggs, soy sauce and tahini just until they form a chunky paste.

In a large bowl, combine the cooled beet mixture and the lentil mixture. Add cooked quinoa, nutritional yeast, ground almonds and ground rolled oats, mix well to combine and let sit for 5 minutes to allow the oats to absorb some moisture.

Heat 1 to 2 tsp of oil in a pan over medium-low heat. Using a greased ice-cream scoop or large serving spoon, add 4 scoops of mixture to the pan and flatten each gently with a spatula to form a patty. Cover and cook for about 8 minutes, or until bottoms are lightly browned and burgers hold together when you slide a spatula under them, then flip and cook on second side for 5 to 6 minutes. I often get two pans going at once to cook all of the patties as quickly as possible, as you have to work in batches. Make sure you keep the heat under medium, and add 1 to 2 tsp of oil to the pan for each batch, otherwise you will likely burn the bottoms.

Tip: These freeze well.

*Makes about 14 large or 18 medium burgers.*

## Simple Chili
*VG, DFO, GFO, CFO*

This is one of my simplest and most popular healthy recipes, and because it's always a hit with visiting kids and serves a crowd, it often gets made for last-minute company. It freezes well, so if you're making a batch, consider doubling it for an easy meal or two down the road. It's so comforting when served with a handful of baked organic corn chips, over brown rice or with a warm Sweet P Biscuit (p. 146).

2 tbsp olive oil
4 garlic cloves, crushed or chopped
1 yellow onion, chopped
2 cups peeled, chopped carrots (about 3 large)
2 cups peeled, cubed sweet potato (about 1 large)
1 can (28 oz/796 mL) crushed tomatoes
1 can (14 oz/398 mL) black beans, rinsed and drained
1 can (14 oz/398 mL) kidney beans, rinsed and drained
2 cups low-sodium vegetable broth
1 cup cooked chickpeas, white beans, black beans or kidney beans — your choice! (canned or freshly cooked)
1 to 2 tbsp chili powder
1 tbsp ground cumin
1 tsp dried dill
1 tsp sea salt
plain Greek yoghurt*

**\*to keep this recipe Cleanstart-friendly, omit the yoghurt**

To make: In a stockpot or Dutch oven, heat oil over medium heat. Cook garlic, onion, carrots and sweet potato about 3 to 5 minutes, until softened. Stir in tomatoes, black beans, kidney beans, broth and chickpeas. Stir in chili powder to taste, cumin, dill and salt.

Reduce heat and simmer for 15 to 20 minutes. Top individual servings with yoghurt, if desired.

Tip: This chili is also very crockpot-friendly. Omit the oil and add all the veggies raw, along with the other ingredients. Stir, then cook on high for 4 hours or low for 8 hours.

*Makes 10 cups.*

## Club Med Veggie Burgers

*V, DF, GF, CF*

Cook these family-friendly, filling patties all in one go and freeze the leftovers.

1 1/4 cups slow-cook rolled oats*
1 onion, peeled and quartered
2 1/2 cups cooked or canned chickpeas, rinsed and drained
4 large eggs
2 tbsp tahini
2 tsp ground cumin
1/2 tsp sea salt
1/3 cup freshly chopped cilantro
1 tbsp grated lemon rind (zest of about 1 lemon)
1 tbsp olive oil

**\* to ensure recipe is gluten-free, use certified gluten-free oats**

To make: Grind rolled oats to a coarse flour in a food processor, then transfer to a bowl and set aside. Chop onion in the food processor, then add chickpeas, eggs, tahini, cumin and salt and purée until mixture has the consistency of a thick, chunky hummus. (If you can still see a few whole chickpeas, that's just fine.) Transfer to a large bowl and add cilantro, lemon rind and ground oats, then stir well and let sit for a couple of minutes so oatmeal can absorb some of the wet mixture.

Heat 1 tsp of oil in skillet on medium-low heat. Using a greased ice-cream scoop or large spoon, add 4 scoops of mixture to the pan and flatten each gently with a spatula to form a patty. Cover and cook for 5 to 7 minutes, or until bottoms are just brown, then flip and cook on second side for 5 to 6 minutes. I often get 2 pans going at once to cook all of the patties as quickly as possible, as you have to work in batches. Make sure you keep the heat under medium, and add another 1 tsp of oil to the pan for each batch, otherwise you will likely burn the bottoms.

Serve topped with Easy Hummus, p. 145, or a little Green Goddess Dressing, p. 143. Leftovers freeze well.

*Makes about 10 large burgers.*

## Spicy Black Bean Burgers
*V, DF, GF, CF*

These are straightforward, tasty, protein-packed burgers. Pre-cook your quinoa to save time and you'll whip these up in less than a half hour. Freeze leftovers for a quick lunch or dinner option. Try topping these with Easy Hummus (p. 145) or Smoky Mayo (p. 144).

3/4 cup slow-cook rolled oats, divided*
1 can (14 oz/398 mL) black beans, rinsed and drained (or 1 1/2 cups cooked)
1 egg
2 tbsp low-sodium soy sauce or tamari
1 tbsp tahini
2 garlic cloves, crushed
2 tsp ground cumin
3/4 tsp chili powder
1/4 tsp cinnamon
1/4 tsp sea salt
1 1/2 cups cooked quinoa
1 cup mashed cooked sweet potato
2 green onions, chopped (white and green parts)
1/2 cup packed fresh cilantro, chopped
1 to 2 tsp olive or coconut oil

**\* to ensure recipe is gluten-free, use certified gluten-free oats**

To make: Grind 1/2 cup of the oats to a coarse flour in food processor, transfer to a bowl and set aside.

Combine beans, egg, soy sauce, tahini, garlic, cumin, chili powder, cinnamon and salt in food processor or blender and pulse until just combined into a chunky mixture. (You should still be able to see some of the beans.) Transfer to a large bowl and add quinoa, sweet potato, green onions and cilantro and mix until combined. Stir in the ground oats and the remaining 1/4 cup whole oats and let mixture sit for 5 minutes.

Heat 1 tsp of oil over medium-low to medium heat in a large pan (or use 2 pans at a time to cook burgers in one batch). Using a greased ice-cream scoop or large serving spoon, add four black bean burgers to the pan and gently flatten. Cover and cook for 7 to 8 minutes per side, until browned and set (you want them to feel solid enough to flip). Check often to ensure bottoms are not burning.

*Makes 8 large burgers.*

# Karmic Buddha Bowls

*VG, DF, GF, CF*

This is one of my most popular recipes, so do yourself a favour and give it a try! You can make the sauce in advance, just give it a shake to recombine before serving, and you can also pre-cook your rice. Or throw some brown rice in the rice cooker about an hour before you prep the veggies and sauce, and you're off to the races!

1 garlic clove, crushed
1/2 cup water
1/4 cup olive oil
1/4 cup nutritional yeast
1/4 cup low-sodium soy sauce or tamari
1/4 cup apple cider vinegar
2 tbsp tahini
2 tsp coconut oil
1 block (454 g) firm organic tofu, cubed*
2 cups grated carrots (about 4 large)**
2 cups grated beets (about 3 to 4)**
2 cups grated red or green cabbage**
Beet greens from beets, above, chopped
1 to 2 cups chopped spinach, kale, bok choy or chard
2 cups cooked brown rice

**\*2 cups pre-cooked cubed chicken breast can be substituted for the tofu**

**\*\*the grater attachment on your food processor makes quick work of this task**

To make: In food processor, combine garlic, water, olive oil, nutritional yeast, soy sauce, vinegar and tahini and blend until smooth. Set sauce aside.

In wok or large frying pan, melt coconut oil over medium heat. Stir-fry tofu until golden. With slotted spoon, remove tofu and set aside.

In the same wok, stir-fry carrots, beets, cabbage, beet greens and spinach until slightly softened, adding a little water to the pan to prevent sticking as needed. Into each of 6 serving bowls, spoon 1/3 cup rice, evenly divide veggie mixture overtop and sprinkle equally with tofu. Top each with about 2 tbsp to 1/4 cup of the sauce, to your own taste.

*Serves 6.*

# Santa Fe Turkey Chili

*DF, GF, VO, CF*

This is a family-friendly, Southwestern-style chili with just a little kick and a hint of lime. If you love your chili hot, dial it up a notch with more chili and smoked paprika. To keep it vegetarian, simply substitute the ground turkey with one more can of beans of your choice — it's just as delicious meat-free! This chili can easily be made in a crockpot — just brown your onions and meat on the stove, then transfer to crockpot, add rest of ingredients and cook on low for 8 hours while you are out.

1/2 tsp olive oil
1 red onion, chopped
3 garlic cloves, crushed
1 lb (454 g) extra-lean ground turkey or chicken*
1 can (28 oz/796 mL) crushed tomatoes
1 can (28 oz/796 mL) diced tomatoes
1 can (14 oz/398 mL) black beans, rinsed (or 1 1/2 cups cooked)
1 can (14 oz/398 mL) kidney beans, rinsed (or 1 1/2 cups cooked)
1 sweet potato, peeled and diced
1 cup organic frozen corn kernels
1 cup low-sodium vegetable or chicken broth
1 tbsp chili powder
1 tbsp ground cumin
1/2 tsp smoked paprika**
1/2 tsp sea salt
2 to 3 tsp grated lime rind (rind of 1 lime)
2 tbsp lime juice

**\*for a vegetarian chili, substitute an additional 14 oz/398 mL can of beans of your choice for the turkey**

**\*\*if you don't like the "smoky" flavour this spice imparts, use regular paprika instead**

To make: In a large pot, heat the olive oil over medium. Cook the onions, garlic and turkey until turkey is browned, then add crushed tomatoes, diced tomatoes, black beans, kidney beans, sweet potato, corn, broth, chili powder, cumin, paprika, salt, lime rind and juice. Bring to a rolling boil then reduce to a low boil, cover and cook until the sweet potato is tender, about 30 to 40 minutes.

This is yummy over brown rice or quinoa or served with organic corn chips and a dollop of Greek yoghurt on top. (Skip the corn chips and yoghurt if you're keeping things dairy-free or following Cleanstart.)

*Makes about 12 cups.*

## Lemony Fish Cakes

*GF, DF, CF*

These are a hit with little and big people — dress them up or down by varying your side dish! Gluten-, dairy- and sugar-free, they're clean comfort food. If you're pressed for time, pre-cook your fish at 350°F for about 18 minutes the night before.

400 to 450 g white fish fillets, pre-cooked
1 cooked sweet potato and/or white potato, mashed
2 green onions, chopped
2 tbsp chopped fresh parsley
2 tsp Dijon mustard
1 tbsp grated lemon rind (or rind of 1 lemon)
3 tbsp lemon juice (or juice of 1 lemon)
1/4 tsp sea salt
1/8 tsp black pepper
2 eggs, beaten
1/2 cup slow-cook rolled oats*
2 tsp olive oil

**\* to ensure recipe is gluten-free, use certified gluten-free oats**

To make: In a large bowl, combine pre-cooked fish, mashed potato, green onions, parsley, mustard, lemon rind and juice, salt and pepper and mash and mix to combine well. Stir in eggs and oats and let sit five minutes.

Heat oil in a large frying pan over medium heat. Form the fish mixture into 8 large, or 14 smaller, cakes and cook in batches for 8 to 10 minutes on each side, until golden brown. These fish cakes freeze well.

*Serves 4 to 5.*

# Lively Lentil Loaf

*V, GF, DF*

Even the thirteen-year-old babysitter likes this one. It's a great alternative to a meat-based main dish, because it's full of protein and has a hearty, slightly spicy flavour.

1 cup slow-cook rolled oats*
2 tbsp olive oil
3 garlic cloves, crushed
1 cup diced mushrooms, any type
3 green onions, chopped
1 medium yellow onion, diced
1 medium potato or sweet potato, peeled and diced
2 small or 1 large carrot, diced
2 ribs celery, diced
1/2 cup low-sodium vegetable broth, divided
3 cups pre-cooked green lentils, divided
3 eggs
1/2 tsp sea salt
1/4 tsp black pepper
1/2 tsp smoked paprika**
1/2 tsp dried thyme
2 cups finely chopped baby spinach

## Sauce

1 cup natural tomato or pasta sauce
1/4 tsp smoked paprika*
1/2 tsp maple syrup
2 tsp yellow mustard
2 tsp apple cider vinegar

**\* to ensure recipe is gluten-free, use certified gluten-free oats**

**\*\*if you don't like the "smoky" flavour this spice imparts, use regular paprika instead**

To make: Grind oats in food processor to a coarse flour, then transfer to bowl and set aside.

In a large saucepan, heat the oil over medium heat. Add the garlic, mushrooms, green and yellow onion, potato, carrot and celery and cook for 5 minutes, stirring. Add 1/4 cup of broth to pan and continue cooking about another 5 minutes or until veggies are softened.

Make the sauce by whisking tomato sauce, paprika, maple syrup, mustard and vinegar together in a medium bowl and set aside.

In the meantime, in a food processor, pulse 1 1/2 cups of the lentils, the remaining 1/4 cup of broth, eggs, salt, pepper, smoked paprika and thyme until a chunky paste forms. Pour into a large bowl, and add remaining lentils, the cooked veggie mixture, chopped spinach and 1/2 of the sauce mixture. Stir to combine and add ground oats. Let sit 5 minutes to allow the oats to absorb some of the liquid, then spread evenly into a greased 8- x 8-inch baking dish. Spread the remaining sauce over the top. Bake in 350°F oven for 50 minutes.

*Serves 6.*

## Creamy Leeks & White Beans with Tarragon

*VG, DF, GF, CF*

Healthy fast food, anyone? This simple, melt-in-your-mouth recipe takes less than 20 minutes to make and can be served over pre-cooked brown rice for a quick, complete meal.

1 tbsp coconut oil
3 to 4 leeks, white parts only, sliced lengthwise, cleaned, and cut into half moons
1/2 tsp sea salt
3 tsp chopped fresh tarragon (or 1 tsp dried, in a pinch)
1/2 tsp dried thyme
1/2 cup unsweetened almond (or cow's) milk
1 can (14 oz/398 mL) white beans, rinsed (or 1 1/2 cups cooked)

To make: Melt the coconut oil in a large pan over medium heat. Add leeks and salt and cook, stirring often, about 10 minutes, until soft. Add tarragon, thyme, milk and beans and cook, stirring, another 5 minutes or until milk is absorbed and beans heated through. Serve warm.

*Serves 4.*

## Don't Falafel the Wagon

*V, GF, DFO, CFO*

You can make this simple dinner in less than half an hour from start to finish. Baked not fried, these falafels are also gluten-free. They freeze well, so consider making a double batch to use during the week. Serve 2 to 3 falafels tucked into a pita half, topped with sliced cucumber, tomato, red onion and a dollop of Tahini Topper for a quick, portable meal.

1/2 cup slow-cook rolled oats, divided*
1 can (14 oz/398 mL) chickpeas, rinsed and drained (or 1 1/2 cups cooked chickpeas)
1/4 cup chopped onion
1/4 cup packed fresh cilantro
1/4 cup packed fresh parsley
1 tbsp tahini
1 tbsp water
1 tsp lemon juice
2 tsp ground cumin
1/4 tsp ground coriander
Pinch chili powder
1/4 tsp sea salt
1/4 tsp aluminum-free baking powder
1 large egg, beaten
1/4 cup crumbled feta cheese (optional**)

## Tahini Topper
1 tbsp lemon juice
3/4 cup plain Greek yoghurt**
1 tbsp tahini
2 to 3 tsp water (or more)
**\*to ensure recipe is gluten-free, use certified gluten-free oats**

**\*\*to keep this recipe dairy-free and Cleanstart-friendly, omit the cheese and skip the Tahini Topper**

To make: In food processor, grind 1/4 cup of oats to a flour. Transfer to large bowl and set aside.

In food processor, combine chickpeas, onion, cilantro, parsley, tahini, water, lemon juice, cumin, coriander, chili powder, salt and baking powder and blend until combined. Stir into bowl with ground oats, along with remaining 1/4 cup whole oats, egg and feta, if using. Let stand for 5 minutes.

With hands, shape into about 18 small balls and transfer to non-stick baking sheet. Flatten slightly. Bake in 400°F oven for 20 minutes, gently turning once halfway through.

In bowl, whisk together Tahini Topper ingredients until smooth, adding enough water to achieve desired consistency.

*Serves 6.*

## Maple-Sage Roasted Chicken Dinner

*DF, GF*

This is an easy to assemble, one-dish dinner and a great way to use up the fall bounty of root veggies. You need just over an hour to roast it all, so be sure to pop it in the oven early enough. If you've got the time (and are really organized) you can boost the flavour by marinating the chicken in the fridge for longer.

8 to 10 cups chopped (into 1.5-inch pieces) root veggies, any combination*
1 onion, quartered and broken into pieces
4 garlic cloves, peeled and sliced in half
2 tsp melted coconut oil
2 tbsp balsamic vinegar
2 tbsp maple syrup
1/4 cup low-sodium chicken or vegetable broth
1 tbsp chopped fresh sage (or 1 tsp dried)
1 tbsp chopped fresh rosemary (or 1 tsp dried)
1/8 tsp sea salt
1/8 tsp black pepper
2 to 3 boneless chicken breasts (enough for your family/group)

**\*sweet potatoes, potatoes, parsnips, carrots, beets, radishes, turnips, squash, kohlrabi and brussels sprouts all work well**

To make: In a large bowl, toss chopped root veggies, onion and garlic with the melted coconut oil until coated evenly.

Transfer to an 11- x 9-inch baking dish and roast at 400°F for 45 minutes.

In the meantime, whisk together balsamic, maple syrup, broth, sage, rosemary, salt and pepper and marinate the chicken in it until it's time to add it to the roasting pan.

At the 45-minute mark, add the chicken and marinade to the veggie mixture and toss to coat. Roast another 25 to 27 minutes or until chicken is cooked through and veggies are tender.

*Serves 5 to 6.*

## Shepherd's Pie with Rosemary Mashed Potatoes

*VG, DF, GF*

Delicious, hearty and satisfying, this will please even the die-hard carnivores at the table. Pre-cook your potatoes and lentils to save time.

### Mashed Potato Base Layer

2 tsp olive oil

2 small or 1 large yellow onion, diced

2 ribs celery, diced

2 carrots, diced

4 cups diced white mushrooms, any type (you'll need about 12 oz of mushrooms)

2 tbsp low-sodium soy or tamari sauce

1 tbsp mirin or cooking wine

1/2 tsp sea salt

1 1/2 tsp smoked paprika*

1 tsp dried thyme

2 cups cooked green lentils**

4 cups finely chopped kale

1 cup green peas (frozen or fresh; if fresh, pre-cook and drain)

1 medium tomato, chopped

1/3 cup chopped fresh parsley

### Mashed Potato Top Layer

6 medium potatoes, coarsely chopped (about 6 cups)

1/2 cups unsweetened almond (or cow's) milk (or more)

1/4 cup nutritional yeast

1 tbsp finely chopped fresh rosemary (or 1 tsp dried)

1 large garlic clove, crushed

1/4 tsp sea salt

1/4 tsp black pepper

To make: In a large saucepan or wok, heat oil over medium heat. Add onions, celery and carrots and cook 7 to 8 minutes or until just softened. Add mushrooms and continue cooking until mushrooms begin to release their juice and veggies are tender. Stir in soy sauce, mirin, salt, paprika, thyme, lentils, kale, peas, tomato and parsley and continue cooking until kale is wilted.

Meanwhile, boil potatoes in a large pot of water until soft. Drain, then transfer to a large bowl and mash. Beat in milk, nutritional yeast, rosemary, garlic, salt and pepper, adding more milk if necessary to provide a creamy, spreadable consistency.

Spread the veggie and lentil mixture evenly into an 11- x 9-inch baking dish, then top with an even layer of the potato mixture. Bake at 350°F for 45 minutes. You can drizzle the top with a little olive oil towards the end of the baking time if you're feeling extra decadent.

*Serves 8.*

**\*if you don't like the "smoky" flavour this spice imparts, use regular paprika instead**

**\*\*either pre-cook 3/4 cup dry green lentils or use canned lentils, drained**

## Oven-Baked Butternut Squash Risotto

*V, GF*

There's no stirring, sweating or standing over the stove for hours with this risotto! This deliciously creamy brown rice dish cooks up in less than an hour, in one pot, with minimal stirring. It's wonderful as a side with grilled meat or veggies or on its own as a comforting, cold-weather main dish.

1 tbsp coconut oil

2 leeks, white & light green parts only, thinly sliced

2 garlic cloves, crushed

1/2 butternut squash, peeled, seeds removed, and cut into 1/2-inch cubes (about 8 cups cubed)

2 cups short-grain brown rice

1 tsp sea salt, divided

1/4 tsp black pepper

1 tsp dried thyme

1 tsp fresh or dried crumbled sage (or 1/2 tsp dried powdered sage)

4 cups low-sodium vegetable broth

3 cups water

1/3 cup grated Asiago or Parmesan cheese

To make: In a large ovenproof Dutch oven, melt the coconut oil over medium heat, then cook the leeks and garlic, stirring, until leeks are slightly softened. Add the squash, rice, 1/2 tsp salt, pepper, thyme and sage and stir for 3 minutes to gently toast the rice. Add the broth and water and increase heat to bring to a rolling boil.

Once boiling, cover and place the Dutch oven into a 425°F oven and bake for 50 minutes or until liquid is absorbed and rice is tender. Remove from oven and gently stir in cheese. The squash will soften and mix in a bit as you do this, but have no fear, this just adds to the dish's creaminess. Add more salt to taste as necessary. I usually add another 1/2 tsp or so.

*Makes 12 cups.*

## This Chalet Chicken

*GF, DF, CF*

Roasting your own whole chicken is economical, straightforward and downright delicious. It's a great habit to cook one on the weekend, then you can carve it up and use it for sandwiches during the week or freeze some for a later date. Even better, while you're at it, roast two! 1 garlic clove, crushed

1 tsp coconut oil, melted
1 tsp poultry seasoning
1/4 tsp salt
3 1/2 lb whole roasting chicken
1 lemon or lime, quartered

To make: In small bowl, stir together garlic, oil, poultry seasoning and salt.

With your fingers, loosen skin on chicken breast and thighs. Rub garlic mixture evenly under skin. Place lemon or lime into cavity. Transfer chicken, breast side up, to a rack set in a roasting pan. Bake at 400°F for about 70 minutes, until meat thermometer inserted into thigh (do not touch bone) registers 180°F.

Let stand for 10 minutes. Remove lemon or lime and skin, then carve.

*Serves 6.*

## Bottomless Chicken Pot Pie

*DF*

Here's a comforting dish for a chilly evening. Dairy-free, packed with veggies and flavour and topped with whole grain biscuits — yum! Don't forget to pre-cook your chicken.

1 tbsp coconut oil
1/2 cup diced celery (about 1 large rib)
1/2 cup chopped leek (about 1 leek, white part only)
1/2 cup diced carrot (about 1 large carrot)
2 cups chopped mushrooms, any type
1 1/2 cups chopped broccoli
1 cup fresh or frozen peas (if frozen, no need to defrost)
2 large cloves garlic, crushed
1 tsp dried thyme
1/2 tsp black pepper
1/4 tsp nutmeg
1 cup packed finely chopped spinach or chard
1/2 cup packed finely chopped fresh parsley
2 cups cooked chicken, shredded or cut into 1/2-inch cubes (about 2 medium boneless breasts)
2 cups low-sodium chicken broth, divided
3 tbsp arrowroot powder (you can use flour in a pinch)
1 cup unsweetened almond (or cow's) milk, divided
1 tbsp Dijon mustard
1/2 tsp sea salt

### Biscuit Topping

2 cups whole wheat flour
1 tbsp baking powder
3/4 tsp sea salt
3 tbsp solid coconut oil
3/4 cup unsweetened almond (or cow's) milk

To make: In a large pan, melt coconut oil over medium heat, then add celery, leek, carrot, mushrooms, broccoli, peas and garlic and cook about 10 to 15 minutes, until veggies are softened. Add thyme, pepper, nutmeg, spinach and parsley and cook another 5 minutes, until spinach is wilted. Transfer mixture to a large bowl and toss in cooked chicken.

While filling is cooking, make biscuits. Combine flour, baking powder and salt in a medium bowl, cut in the coconut oil with two knives or a pastry cutter, then stir in milk until well combined. Roll out gently on a well-floured surface to about 3/4-inch thick, and cut out about 12 biscuits with the edge of a 3-inch diameter drinking glass or circular cookie cutter.

In the same large pan, bring 1 cup of chicken broth to a boil, then reduce heat to low. In a small bowl, whisk arrowroot with 1/2 cup of almond milk, then slowly add to heated chicken broth, whisking continuously. Mixture will thicken considerably. Slowly whisk in the rest of the broth, milk, mustard and salt until well combined.

Add the filling back to the pan and combine well with the sauce, then transfer mixture to an 11- x 9-inch baking dish. Top with an evenly distributed layer of biscuits. Bake at 425°F for 17 to 20 minutes, or until biscuit top is a light golden colour. Let sit 10 minutes before serving.

*Serves 6 to 8.*

## Lentil Sloppy Joes
*VG, DFO*

Comfort food epitomized. So good, I swear you won't miss the meat!

1 tbsp olive oil
1 onion, chopped
1 garlic clove, crushed
1 green bell pepper, diced
1 rib celery, diced
8 oz (227 g) mushrooms, diced
1 1/2 cups cooked green lentils
1/2 cup chopped walnuts
1 can (28 oz/796 mL) crushed tomatoes
2 tbsp maple syrup
1 tbsp lime juice
2 tsp apple cider vinegar
1 1/2 tsp ground cumin
1 1/2 tsp chili powder
1 tsp dried dill
1 tsp oregano
1 tsp smoked paprika*
3/4 tsp sea salt
1/4 tsp black pepper
6 to 8 slices Ezekiel sprouted grain or 100% whole grain bread
Asiago or Parmesan cheese, to garnish (optional**)

**\*to keep this recipe dairy-free, omit the cheese**

**\*\*if you don't like the "smoky" flavour this spice imparts, use regular paprika instead**

To make: In a very large saucepan or wok, heat the olive oil over medium heat, then add onion and garlic and cook until onion softened, about 5 minutes. Add bell pepper, celery, and mushrooms and sauté about another 10 minutes, until mushrooms begin to release their liquid.

Add lentils, walnuts, tomatoes, maple syrup, lime juice, vinegar, cumin, chili, dill, oregano, paprika, salt and pepper and stir well. Heat through then reduce heat and simmer about 10 minutes. Serve over 1 or 2 slices of Ezekiel sprouted grain or whole grain toast and top with a little grated Asiago or Parmesan.

*Makes about 5 cups.*
*Serves 6 to 7 (3/4 cup Sloppy Joe mixture per serving).*

# Crockpot Chicken Fajitas

*GFO, DFO, CFO*

This is a really easy way to serve up delicious, juicy fajitas on a busy weeknight. The meat and veggies cook while you're out, so you can assemble your wraps or rice bowls quickly at dinnertime. Don't forget to pre-cook some brown rice, or make a batch of Wholly Homemade Tortillas (p. 147).

2 medium-sized boneless, skinless chicken breasts
1 red bell pepper, sliced
1 orange bell pepper, sliced
1 yellow bell pepper, sliced
1 red onion, sliced
2 tbsp lime juice
1 tsp honey*
2 garlic cloves, minced
2 tsp chili powder
1 tsp ground cumin
1 tsp paprika
1/2 tsp sea salt
1/8 tsp cayenne pepper
plain yoghurt, salsa and fresh cilantro, to garnish*
pre-cooked brown rice or whole grain tortillas, for serving*

**\*to keep this recipe dairy-free, omit the yoghurt; to keep it gluten-free, serve over brown rice or use gluten-free tortillas; to keep it Cleanstart-friendly, omit the honey and yoghurt and serve over brown rice.**

To make: Place chicken breasts in the bottom of the slow cooker, topping with peppers and onion. In a small bowl, whisk together lime juice, honey, garlic, chili powder, cumin, paprika, salt and cayenne, then pour mixture over veggies and chicken. Cook on low for 6 hours or high for 3 to 4 hours.

Once cooked, chicken will shred easily with a fork.

To serve, top either rice or a tortilla with shredded chicken and veggies, salsa, a dollop of plain yoghurt and some freshly chopped cilantro.

*Makes about 2 cups shredded chicken and 1 cup cooked veggies.*

**Tip: If you are serving more than 5, just add an extra chicken breast and bell pepper to the crockpot; it will still have plenty of flavour.**

*Serves 5.*

# Mama's Little Helper

*GFO*

In the interest of full disclosure, let me say this: I have no idea what Hamburger Helper tastes like. But I've seen it, and I've seen the ingredient list, and this is my healthy, tasty homemade version. My son loves this so much he has learned to make it from start to finish himself, so now we jokingly refer to him as "Mama's Little Helper."

This is an easy crockpot recipe you can also make on the stove.

1 lb (454 g) lean ground beef, preferably grass-fed and naturally-raised
1 onion, chopped
2 garlic cloves, crushed
2 cups finely chopped fresh or frozen kale
3 carrots, peeled and chopped
1 can (28 oz/796 mL) diced tomatoes
2 cups unsweetened almond (or cow's) milk
1 cup water
1/3 cup nutritional yeast
1 tsp chili powder
1 tsp sea salt
1/2 tsp smoked or regular paprika
1 1/2 cups dry 100% whole grain macaroni*
1/2 cup plain, non-fat Greek yoghurt
1/3 cup shredded white cheddar cheese

* To keep this recipe gluten-free, use gluten-free macaroni or other pasta

To make: Crockpot method: In a pan on the stovetop, brown the beef and drain off any extra fat. In a crockpot, combine browned beef with onion, garlic, kale, carrots, tomatoes, almond milk, water, nutritional yeast, chili powder, salt and paprika. Stir to combine and cook on high for about 3 hours (or low for 6 hours).

After 3 hours on high, add dry macaroni and let mixture cook another half hour or until noodles are tender. (If cooking on low, cook your macaroni separately, drain and add to crockpot.) Stir in yoghurt and cheese until well blended, then remove from heat and serve.

Stovetop method: Brown beef in a large pot and then add onion, garlic, kale, carrots, tomatoes, almond milk, water, nutritional yeast, chili powder, salt, and paprika. Bring to a boil, then simmer until veggies are tender. Add pasta and cook to desired tenderness, then stir in yoghurt and cheese.

*Makes about 11 cups.*

## Mexican Spaghetti Squash Bake

*V, GF*

This creamy and comforting casserole is also super healthy — and no one will even miss the pasta! Pre-roast your squash the night or morning before for quicker delivery on a busy evening. Serve as a vegetarian main course, or as a side dish with grilled chicken or fish.

1 large or 1 1/2 small spaghetti squash
1 tbsp olive oil
1 cup chopped red onion
3 garlic cloves, crushed
1 green bell pepper, diced
1 can (28 oz/796 mL) whole tomatoes, drained and broken up with a fork
1 can (14 oz/398 mL) black beans, rinsed well (or 1 1/2 cups cooked)
2 tbsp lime juice
1/2 cup plain yoghurt
1/4 cup chopped fresh cilantro
1 tbsp ground cumin
1 tsp chili powder
1 tsp dried oregano
1/2 tsp sea salt
1/2 cup cubed feta cheese (or shredded white cheddar cheese)
1/3 cup grated Asiago or Parmesan cheese (optional)

To make: Cut squash lengthwise, remove seeds, puncture skin with a knife tip then place cut-side down on a parchment-lined or lightly greased baking sheet. Bake at 375°F for 35 to 40 minutes or until skin is soft and flesh scoops away fairly easily. Let cool a bit to make it easier to handle.

In the meantime, heat oil in a large pan over medium heat. Add the onion, garlic and green pepper and cook for about 10 minutes or until pepper softens. Remove from heat and stir in tomatoes, beans, lime juice, yoghurt, cilantro, cumin, chili powder, oregano, salt and feta.

Lightly grease an 11- x 9-inch baking dish. Scoop the flesh from the squash halves into the pan (your yield should be about 6 cups roasted squash), then pour the veggie mixture over top and stir to thoroughly combine. Distribute evenly in pan and top with grated Asiago cheese, if using. Bake at 375°F for 20 minutes or until just bubbling.

*Serves 8 as a main course.*

## Zucchini Noodles with Avocado Pesto

*VO, GF, VGO, DFO*

Zucchini noodles, or as we like to call them, "zoodles," are a satisfying, non-gluten pasta alternative when topped with marinara sauce and meatballs or a decadent creamy sauce like this Avocado Pesto and some grilled chicken. You'll need a spiralizer or julienne peeler to make the zoodles, which you can find at your local kitchen store.

2 to 4 medium zucchini, washed with ends trimmed*
2 cups fresh spinach
1 avocado, pitted and peeled
1 cup packed fresh basil
1/4 cup walnuts or pecans
1/4 cup grated Asiago or Parmesan cheese (optional**)
3 small garlic cloves, crushed
2 tbsp lemon juice
1/4 tsp black pepper
1/8 tsp sea salt
1/4 cup olive oil
grilled chicken, enough to serve your group**

**\*2 medium zucchini will serve 2, 4 zucchini will serve 4**

**\*\* to keep this recipe dairy-free, omit the cheese or substitute 1 tbsp nutritional yeast; to keep it vegetarian, omit the chicken; to keep it vegan, omit the cheese, or substitute 1 tbsp nutritional yeast, and omit the chicken**

To make: Using a spiralizer or julienne peeler, turn your zucchini into "noodles." If using a julienne peeler, you'll have to pull the noodles apart with your fingers after peeling a strip.

Add spinach, avocado, basil, walnuts, Asiago (if using), garlic, lemon juice, pepper and salt to food processor and blend until smooth. While continuing to blend, add oil slowly until a thick, smooth sauce results. In a large bowl, toss the sauce (or half of the sauce if you are only serving 2) with the zoodles and let sit for 5 minutes or so, which will soften the raw zucchini up nicely.

Top each serving with 4 oz grilled chicken. Leftovers can be frozen.

*Serves 2 to 4. Makes about 1 1/2 cups of sauce.*

## Taco Tuesday Two Ways

*VO*

Quick tacos two ways: fish or vegetarian. Both are healthy and delicious, with the same zesty cilantro-lime yoghurt and cabbage & avocado slaw. You choose! You'll need 10 small or 6 large whole grain soft tortillas. Try making my four-ingredient Wholly Homemade Tortillas (p. 147) and you might never go back to store-bought!

### Way 1 — Tofu Filling

2 tbsp olive oil, divided
3/4 cup chopped onion
2 garlic cloves, crushed
1 block (454 g) firm organic tofu, crumbled
1 1/2 tbsp chili powder
1 1/2 tsp ground cumin
1/4 tsp black pepper
1/4 tsp smoked paprika*
1 tbsp maple syrup

To make: Heat 1 tbsp oil in large pan over medium heat, then add onion and garlic and cook until softened. Add tofu, chili powder, cumin, pepper, paprika and maple syrup and stir well to coat evenly. Cook another 5 minutes, or until tofu is heated through.

### Way 2 — Fish Filling

1 lb (454 g) white fish of your choice
1 tbsp lime juice
1 tbsp maple syrup
1 tsp olive oil
1 garlic clove, crushed
1 tsp chili powder
1/2 tsp ground cumin
1/4 tsp smoked paprika*

*if you don't like the "smoky" flavour this spice imparts, use regular paprika instead

To make: Place fish in a baking dish. In a small bowl combine lime juice, maple syrup, oil, garlic, chili powder, cumin and paprika, then spread evenly over fish. Bake at 350°F for 20 to 25 minutes or until fish is opaque.

### Cilantro-Lime Yoghurt

3/4 cup plain Greek yoghurt
1 1/2 tsp grated lime rind
1 tbsp lime juice
1/8 tsp salt
1/4 tsp maple syrup
1 1/2 tbsp chopped fresh cilantro

To make: In a small bowl combine yoghurt, lime rind and juice, salt, maple syrup and cilantro. Set aside.

### Cabbage & Avocado Slaw

1/2 cup chopped cabbage, any type
1 large tomato, chopped
1/2 an avocado, chopped
squeeze of lime juice (optional)

To make: In a bowl, combine cabbage, tomato, avocado and lime juice, if using. Set aside.

Assemble tortillas by topping centre of each with some tofu or fish filling then some slaw, and topping with 1 tbsp or so of Cilantro-Lime Yoghurt.

*Makes enough for 10 small or 6 large tortillas.*
*Serves 6.*

## Stir It Up!

*VG, DF, GF, CFO*

Easy and versatile, these tasty stir-fry sauces will pair well with any random veggies hiding in the back corners of your fridge. Sometimes I'm too lazy to mix them up outside of the wok, and just make a well in the centre of the veggies, throw in the sauce ingredients and toss them with the veggies. Less sophisticated, but it does the trick!

This recipe serves 6, but if you are only cooking for 1 or 2, you can easily reduce the protein and veggies accordingly and reserve the extra sauce for a future meal.

2 tsp coconut oil, divided
1 block (454 g) tofu or 2 medium chicken breasts, cubed
8 cups chopped mixed veggies of your choice (such as cabbage, bok choy, broccoli, carrots, celery, bell peppers, chard, beet greens)

## Simple Stir-fry Sauce

1/4 cup low-sodium soy sauce or tamari
1/4 cup apple cider vinegar
2 tbsp tahini
1/3 cup nutritional yeast
1 garlic clove, crushed
1/4 cup water, and more to thin as needed

## Nutty Lime Sauce

1/3 cup natural almond or peanut butter*
2 tsp low-sodium soy sauce or tamari
2 tsp apple cider vinegar
2 tbsp lime juice
1 garlic clove, crushed
1/2 cup water

**\*to keep this recipe Cleanstart-friendly, use almond butter**

To make: In a wok or large frying pan, over medium-high heat, cook the protein of your choice (tofu or chicken) in 1 tsp coconut oil until chicken is cooked through or tofu is golden, then remove from heat and set aside.

In the same pan, over medium heat, stir-fry the mixed chopped veggies in the remaining 1 tsp of coconut oil. Add a little water to prevent burning, then cover and cook until vegetables reach desired tenderness.

In the meantime, whisk up your sauce of choice in a separate bowl. Add cooked protein back to pan, then stir in the sauce and bring to a low boil. Reduce heat and simmer mixture for a couple of minutes to thicken, adding a little more water if it gets too thick.

*Serves 6.*

## Easy Spelt Veggie Pizza

*V*

Be a dinner hero — there's no need to cut out pizza night! This super-quick spelt thin crust is topped with homemade or jarred natural tomato sauce, loads of chopped veggies and just enough cheese to satisfy your cravings and still keep you on track!

## Crust

2 cups spelt flour
1 1/2 tsp quick rise or instant yeast
1/2 tsp sea salt
1 tsp dried oregano
1 tsp dried basil
1 garlic clove, crushed
2/3 cup warm water
1 tbsp honey
1 tbsp olive oil

## Toppings

3/4 to 1 cup jarred (or homemade) natural tomato or pasta sauce
2 cups spinach, chopped
2 cups chopped veggies of choice (tomatoes, peppers, mushrooms, artichoke hearts, olives, etc.)
1 cup shredded white mozzarella, old cheddar or feta, or some combination of these

To make: Preheat oven to 425°F. Lightly spray or brush a large baking sheet or pizza pan with oil.

Combine the flour, yeast, salt, oregano, basil and garlic in a large bowl and mix well. Add the water, honey and oil and mix until well combined and a ball of dough forms (you'll probably need to get your hands in there).

Cover the bowl with a clean, damp towel and let it rise on the stovetop, with the preheating oven door open just a crack, for about 10 minutes.

On a well-floured surface, knead the dough for about 3 minutes, adding more flour if it's sticky. Punch the ball down to form a flat disc, then roll out the dough until it's large enough to cover the pizza pan. (I like it quite thin, covering almost the whole of a large cookie sheet.) Stretch the dough up the sides of the pan, or roll the edges down, to form a small crust around the edge.

Add toppings and cheese and bake at 425°F for about 20 minutes, or until crust is crispy and brown.

*Serves 5.*

# CHAPTER 16

# *Salad Dressings & Sauces*

## Creamy Avocado Dressing
*VG, DF, GF, CF*

This decadent dressing is packed with healthy fat and flavour.

1 avocado, peeled and pitted
1 small shallot, quartered
1 small garlic clove, crushed
2 tbsp apple cider vinegar
2 tsp lemon or lime juice
2 tbsp fresh cilantro (or 2 tsp dried)
1/2 tsp ground cumin
1/4 tsp chili powder
1/4 tsp sea salt
1/2 cup water (or more as needed)

To make: In a food processor or blender, combine avocado, shallot, garlic, vinegar, lemon juice, cilantro, cumin, chili powder and salt and blend until smooth. Add water slowly, while blending, until dressing reaches creamy consistency.

Transfer to a sealed jar and store in the fridge for up to 5 days, adding water to thin as necessary before each use.

*Makes about 1 1/2 cups or 24 table-spoons.*

## Beat the Band Balsamic

*VG, DF, GF*

Store-bought salad dressings are full of suspect ingredients like unhealthy oils, artificial flavours and preservatives. Simple and delicious, this homemade dressing shakes up in one jar and keeps for 5 to 7 days — so make a batch and you're good to go for lunches all week long.

1/2 cup olive oil
2 tbsp lime juice (about the juice of one lime)
1/4 cup balsamic vinegar
1 tbsp tahini
2 tbsp water
1 tsp Dijon mustard
1 tsp maple syrup
1 clove crushed garlic

To make: Combine oil, lime juice, vinegar, tahini, water, mustard, maple syrup and garlic in a jar and shake until well combined. Store unused portion in fridge. When using refrigerated dressing, let it warm to room temperature and shake it gently to recombine, adding a little more water if necessary to thin.

*Makes about 1 1/4 cups or 20 tablespoons.*

## Berry Balsamic

*VG, DF, GF*

This is an easy, sweet salad dressing even kids will love. It's perfect over a summery spinach or arugula salad with tomatoes and pecans or walnuts.

1 cup strawberries (defrosted if frozen)
3 tbsp balsamic vinegar
1 tsp maple syrup (or 2 pitted medjool dates, chopped)
1/8 tsp sea salt
1/8 tsp black pepper
1/4 cup olive oil
1 to 2 tbsp water (optional, add if it's too thick or thickens in fridge )

To make: In a food processor or high-powered blender, purée berries, balsamic, maple syrup (or dates), salt and pepper. Slowly add the olive oil while blending to combine until a creamy dressing forms, slowly adding water as necessary to thin. Store in an airtight jar in the fridge. If dressing thickens in the fridge, add a little more water and shake to recombine before using.

*Makes about 1 1/4 cups or 20 tablespoons.*

## Green Goddess Dressing

*VG, DF, GF, CF*

My most popular salad dressing, this might just single-handedly change the way you feel about salad! This tangy, creamy, dairy-free concoction is downright addictive! Don't skimp: it's totally worth picking up fresh parsley and cilantro. Dried herbs just don't cut it in this one. To make a thicker dip instead, stir in a little plain Greek yoghurt.

2 tbsp lime juice
3 tbsp tahini
1/4 cup packed fresh parsley
1/4 cup packed fresh cilantro
1 green onion, chopped
1 tbsp low-sodium soy or tamari sauce
2 tbsp apple cider vinegar
1/4 tsp black pepper
1/8 to 1/4 tsp sea salt
2 tbsp olive oil

To make: In a food processor, combine lime juice, tahini, parsley, cilantro, green onion, soy sauce, vinegar, pepper and 1/8 tsp salt and blend until smooth. Continue to blend, slowly adding the olive oil until well combined and more salt as needed to taste. Store leftovers in fridge.

*Makes about 3/4 cup or 12 tablespoons.*

## Sesame-Maple Vinaigrette

*VG, DF, GF*

Shake up this sweet Asian dressing in a jar and it's ready. Tangy and versatile, it livens up even the simplest of salads.

2 tsp toasted sesame oil
2 tsp maple syrup
1/4 cup balsamic vinegar
1/4 cup olive oil
1/8 tsp sea salt
1/8 tsp black pepper
1 garlic clove, crushed

To make: Combine sesame oil, maple syrup, vinegar, oil, salt, pepper and garlic in a jar and shake until smooth. Store leftovers in fridge, adding a little water to thin if necessary and shaking before each use.

*Makes about 2/3 cup or 10 tablespoons.*

## Smoky Mayo

*V, GF*

This is the all-purpose condiment you've been looking for — it's great on veggie burgers, meat burgers, sandwiches or as a dip, and it's so much healthier than the creamier processed alternatives. Go ahead, pile it on!

1/2 cup plain Greek yoghurt (non-fat or 2%)
1 tbsp Dijon mustard
1 tbsp tahini
1 tbsp apple cider vinegar
1 tsp ground cumin
1/2 tsp smoked paprika*
pinch of sea salt

**\*if you don't like the "smoky" flavour this spice imparts, use regular paprika instead**

To make: Whisk together yoghurt, mustard, tahini, vinegar, cumin, paprika and salt until well blended. Refrigerate leftovers in a sealed container.

*Makes about 3/4 cup or 12 tablespoons.*

# CHAPTER 17

## Snacks & Sweets

### Easy Hummus
*VG, DF, GF, CF*

You might never buy hummus again. You can whip up a batch of this during a TV commercial break, it's that easy! Freeze a batch in an ice-cube tray, then take a frozen cube to work in a small container and it will be defrosted by lunchtime in the perfect portion size to eat with veggies or pita, or as the spread in a whole grain veggie sandwich.

1 can (14 oz/398 mL) chickpeas, well rinsed (or 1 1/2 cups cooked chickpeas)
1/3 cup tahini
2 to 4 tbsp water
3 tbsp lemon juice
1 to 2 garlic cloves
2 tsp ground cumin
1 tsp salt

To make: Combine in chickpeas, tahini, water (start with 2 tbsp), lemon juice, garlic (start with 1 clove), cumin and salt in food processor and blend, adding more water as needed to reach desired consistency and more garlic as needed to taste.

*Makes about 2 cups.*

## Sweet P Biscuits

*VG, DF*

These biscuits are just a little sweet and a lot tasty. They take only a few minutes to assemble and less than 20 minutes to bake, so they make a perfect last-minute side to any meal.

2 cups whole wheat or spelt flour
2 tsp aluminum-free baking powder
1/2 tsp pumpkin pie spice*
1/4 tsp sea salt
1/4 cup solid coconut oil
1 cup well-cooked, mashed sweet potato (about 1 medium potato)**
1 tbsp unsweetened applesauce
1 tbsp maple syrup
1/3 cup unsweetened almond (or cow's) milk

**\*If you don't have premixed pumpkin pie spice, you can make your own by combining 4 tbsp cinnamon, 4 tsp ground nutmeg, 4 tsp ground ginger and 3 tsp allspice. Store remainder in an airtight jar.**

**\*\*To cook the sweet potato, poke the unpeeled skin of the sweet potato with a fork in a few places and microwave it for 5 to 7 minutes on high, turning once, or roast at 400°F in the oven for about 1 hour.**

To make: In a medium bowl, combine flour, baking powder, pumpkin pie spice and salt. Cut in the coconut oil with a pastry cutter or two knives until mixture resembles fine crumbs with a few larger pieces.

In a smaller bowl, stir together the sweet potato, applesauce, maple syrup and almond milk, then add the wet to the dry ingredients and mix until well combined (don't be afraid to get your hands in there!).

On a lightly floured surface, roll the dough out to 1 inch thick and cut out 10 to 11 biscuits using the mouth of a 2.5-inch diameter drinking glass or round cookie cutter of the same size. If you roll the dough out too thin, your biscuits won't rise nicely.

Place on a baking sheet, with edges of the biscuits just touching each other (this helps them rise better) and bake at 400°F for 16 to 17 minutes, until just golden brown.

*Makes 10 to 11 biscuits.*

# Wholly Homemade Tortillas

*VG, DF*

This is a very basic, foolproof whole wheat tortilla recipe. So much cheaper than buying pre-packaged tortillas, and instead of the usual mammoth list of unpronounceable ingredients in the commercial varieties, these have just 4 simple ingredients.

2 1/4 cups whole wheat flour (or 2 1/2 cups spelt flour)
1/2 tsp sea salt
3 tbsp + 1 tsp olive oil
3/4 cup very warm water

To make: In a medium bowl, mix together flour and salt. Add olive oil and mix with hands until combined (dough will be dry and crumbly). Add the water and continue to mix with hands, kneading in bowl or on counter for a couple of minutes until you can form dough into a nice ball. Cover bowl and let sit 20 to 25 minutes.

Preheat a dry cast iron pan to medium or a non-stick pan to medium-high. (I find a slightly higher temperature is necessary if you aren't using cast iron.)

Divide dough equally into 8 balls by rolling dough into a log, dividing in half with a knife, then dividing each half into 4 equal portions. On a well-floured surface, use a rolling pin to roll each ball as thin as you can (almost paper thin), until you get about an 8-inch diameter to the tortilla. The easiest way to do this is to flatten the ball into a disc with your palm, roll it out, flip it over and roll it out again, and repeat until you get to an 8-inch diameter.

Place 1 tortilla in preheated pan and allow to cook for approximately 1 minute or until bottom is lightly browned and bubbles form on top. Using tongs, turn tortilla over to brown on second side for approximately 30 to 45 seconds more, taking care not to burn the tortilla, then transfer to a plate. Repeat process with each ball of dough.

Cover tortillas with towel to keep warm and moist until serving. Tortillas can be frozen or stored in an airtight container in the fridge. If they are stiff when removed from fridge, warm them slightly to make them more pliable.

*Makes 8 tortillas.*

## Cocoa-Nut Lime Power Balls

*VG, DF, GF*

These are perfectly sweet, simple chocolate truffles with a hint of lime. Wonderful for a pre- or post-workout snack or as a sweet treat with a cup of tea (or a glass of red), these balls are free of added sugars, dairy and gluten, and full of healthy fat. They freeze well, which is helpful if you can't eat just one — out of sight, out of mind!

1 1/2 cups cashews (raw or roasted)
1 1/2 cups pitted medjool dates*
1/3 cup unsweetened coconut
1/3 cup cocoa
1 tsp grated lime rind (about 1 lime)
2 tbsp lime juice

*If your dates are dry, soak them in hot water for a few minutes to moisten and plump them up, then drain them well.

To make: In a food processor, blend cashews to a coarse flour. Add dates, coconut, cocoa, lime rind and juice and continue to blend until well combined. You may have to stop the processor and move the mixture around a bit with a spoon then continue blending to get it well combined. The mixture may seem a little dry, but it should bind together when you roll it into balls. If it doesn't, add a tablespoon of water to the food processor and pulse to combine.

Roll the mixture into 1-inch balls (approximately 1 tbsp of mixture per ball). You can roll each ball in unsweetened shredded coconut for a fancier end product if you like. Refrigerate at least one hour before serving.

*Makes 30 balls.*

## Chocolate Chili Avocado Pudding
*VG, DF, GF*

This dairy-free dessert is full of healthy fat and protein and just sweet enough. The cinnamon, chili and cayenne provide a little gourmet flair. Impress your crowd, then ask them to identify the secret ingredients — they'll never guess! It's rich, so a little goes a long way — I like to serve it in shot-sized glasses.

4 pitted medjool dates*
2 ripe avocados
1/4 cup maple syrup
1/4 cup unsweetened almond milk (or cow's milk)
2 tsp vanilla
1/2 cup cocoa
1/2 tsp cinnamon
1/4 tsp chili powder
1/8 tsp cayenne pepper

*If your dates are dry, soak them in hot water for a few minutes to moisten and plump them up, then drain them well.

To make: In a food processor, process the dates until they form a smooth paste. Add avocados, maple syrup, almond milk, vanilla, cocoa, cinnamon, chili power and cayenne and blend until a very smooth consistency results. (You may need to scrape the sides of the food processor's bowl once or twice.)

*Makes 2 cups. Serves 6 with 1/3 cup portions.*

## Dark Chocolate Chip Banana Bread
*V, DFO*

This healthier banana bread is moist and sweet and the dark chocolate chips totally hit the spot when a craving calls. No refined sugar, 100 per cent whole grain, no dairy, high in fibre and lots of healthy fat: it's a no-guilt indulgence. Make a cup of tea, put your feet up and enjoy!

3 ripe bananas, mashed
2 eggs, beaten
1/2 cup maple syrup
1/2 tsp vanilla extract
2 cups whole wheat or spelt flour
1/4 cup ground flax seeds
1 tbsp chia seeds
1 tsp aluminum-free baking powder
3/4 tsp sea salt
1/4 tsp cinnamon
1/3 cup of dark chocolate chips, or 1/3 of a dark chocolate bar, chopped*

**\*to keep recipe completely dairy-free, use vegan chocolate chips or avoid milk products in your chocolate ingredients**

To make: Lightly grease or line a loaf pan with parchment paper.

In a large bowl, stir together bananas, eggs, maple syrup, vanilla, flour, flax, chia, baking powder, salt, cinnamon and chocolate chips until combined. Spread evenly in loaf pan and bake at 350°F for 55 to 60 minutes, or until top is golden and toothpick inserted in it comes out clean.

*Serves 14.*

# Homemade Almond Milk or Cream

*VG, DF, GF*

If you think making your own almond milk is an involved and tedious process, think again. It's actually very straightforward and the results are so worth it. I especially love making the thicker almond cream because it takes my morning coffee to a whole new level. You can use a cheesecloth in the straining process, but a small investment in a reusable nut-milk bag from your local health food store is also well worth it.

1 cup raw almonds
2 or 4 cups water (use 2 for cream or 4 for milk)
4 or 5 pitted medjool dates (use 4 for cream or 5 for milk)
1/4 tsp cinnamon (optional)
1/2 tsp natural vanilla extract (optional)

To make: Soak almonds in a bowl overnight (use enough water to cover them by an inch or so). The next day, drain almonds and put them in a blender with either 2 or 4 cups of water, depending on whether you are making cream or milk. Blend for about two minutes, then add the dates (and cinnamon and/or vanilla if using) and blend again until smooth.

Place a mesh strainer over a large bowl. Place the nut-milk bag or cheesecloth into the strainer and slowly pour the contents of the blender into the bag or cloth. Let the liquid drain through on its own, letting gravity do the job, or squeeze the cloth or bag to speed up the process.

Once fully drained, put the milk or cream into a sealed jar or container and refrigerate for up to 3 to 4 days. The pulp can be dried and used in baking.

*Makes between 2 to 4 cups.*

## Harvest Crockpot Applesauce
*VG, DF, GF*

Honestly, is there anything dreamier than the smell of cooking apples with cinnamon and vanilla? This applesauce is so good, you feel like you're indulging in something far less healthy. It's the perfect real food dessert for the whole family.

14 to 16 medium to large apples
1 1/2 tsp pumpkin pie spice*
1/4 cup maple syrup (optional)
1/2 tsp vanilla extract

**\*If you don't have premixed pumpkin pie spice, you can make your own by combining 4 tbsp cinnamon, 4 tsp ground nutmeg, 4 tsp ground ginger and 3 tsp allspice. Store remainder in an airtight jar.**

To make: Peel, core and cut the apples into chunks (aim for about 14 cups of cut apples) then toss into your crockpot. Add pumpkin pie spice and maple syrup (it's optional, depending on the sweetness of the apples you are using, but it does give the applesauce a lovely dessert-like flavour).

Cook on high for 4 to 4 1/2 hours until apples are very soft, then add vanilla and mash with a potato masher or fork.

*Makes about 6 cups.*

## "Nice" Cream 2 Ways
*VG, DF, GF*

This healthy ice cream alternative is sugar- and dairy-free, hence the name. Cut up your ripe bananas before they brown and throw them into the freezer in a container, labelling how many are in each container. The Strawberry Banana is sweet and refreshing, and it probably goes without saying that the Chocolate Peanut Butter is just downright divine.

### Strawberry Banana
2 bananas, cut into chunks and frozen
1 cup frozen strawberries
1/2 cup unsweetened coconut or almond milk
1/2 tsp pure vanilla extract

### Chocolate Peanut Butter
4 bananas, cut into chunks and frozen
1 tsp maple syrup
1/4 cup natural peanut butter
1/2 cup unsweetened coconut or almond milk
(start with 1/2 cup, adding more if necessary)
1 tsp vanilla
1/4 cup cocoa

To make: Blend banana chunks first until smooth in a food processor or good quality blender. You will have to stop, stir and restart the processor a couple of times to do this. Once bananas have formed a thick, smooth paste, add the rest of the ingredients and process until smooth. This melts quickly, so serve *immediately* or pop into freezer until you are ready to eat. It will need to soften at room temperature for a few minutes if you refreeze it.

*Serves 4.*

## Dipped & Salted Truffles

*VG, DF, GF*

These are easy to make, delectable and look way fancier than they are. Does it get any better than that? With no cooking involved, your kids can make these even at a young age with some basic supervision. Keep them in the freezer, and you'll always have a sweet, real food treat when you need one, whether you're serving it with a glass of milk or a glass of red.

2 cups pitted medjool dates*
2 cups raw nuts, any variety and combination (try peanuts, almonds or cashews)
1/4 tsp sea salt
2 tbsp cocoa
1 tbsp coconut oil, melted
1 tsp maple syrup
coarse sea salt for sprinkling

*If your dates are dry, soak them in hot water for a few minutes to moisten and plump them up, then drain them well.

To make: In a food processor, blend dates until well puréed. Add nuts and salt and blend again until you get a chunky mixture that you can form easily with your hands. Roll into about 30 small balls (about 1 inch in diameter) using the palms of your hands.

In a small bowl, whisk cocoa into melted coconut oil and maple syrup until it forms a chocolate sauce.

Using a toothpick or skewer, pick up each ball and dip the top half in chocolate sauce, then place ball on plate, chocolate side up. Sprinkle the tops with a touch of coarse sea salt.

Freeze until sauce hardens. Eat chilled and store the leftovers in the freezer.

*Makes 30 balls.*

# PART 4
# TOOLS FOR
# SUCCESS

# CHAPTER 18

## Support and Tools, or "How to Become a Real Food Ninja"

What follows is your real food ninja tool kit — in it you'll find all the key information and tips you need to get this transition to real food done, and done right. Follow my simple strategies for planning, shopping and cooking and before you know it, you too will be a real food ninja.

## STEP 1: BECOME A MEAL-PLANNING NINJA

### Why does meal planning matter?

- It will save you money. In fact, it's the key to eating healthily on a budget.

- It will make grocery shopping quick and painless.

- It will ensure variety in your family's food.

- It will reduce waste.

- It will significantly reduce the amount of processed and convenience food your family eats.

- Most important, it can single-handedly preserve your sanity.

### How to become a meal-planning ninja:

- Get a template for a week's worth of planning. You can download the one I use with my clients for free at **www.formaclorimerbooks.ca/ realfood/mealplan.pdf.** Look at your family calendar and note any activities or events that will make it difficult to cook certain meals or for certain family members to eat with the rest of the family. Record these on your meal planner.

- Go through a healthy recipe book, like this one, and choose some simple meals to try on the days you will have time to cook from scratch. Add these to your planner.

- Don't waste. Check your freezer and pantry. Do you have any foods that need to be used? Incorporate them into this week's plan!

- Don't reinvent the wheel at every meal. At least half of your dinner options should be recipes you've tried before with success.

- Don't regularly cook meals with extravagant or out-of-season ingredients that are going to be costly and difficult to find. Keep it simple.

- On days when you know you will be rushed, either pencil in a healthy fast food option (see my list, page 169) or choose a recipe you can make in advance and freeze, making a note on the planner that you need to take it out to defrost that morning.

- Fill in breakfasts and lunches, making use of leftovers from dinners the night before, and note anywhere you think you might need to double up on a recipe to provide enough for the next day or evening.

- Include a list of family snacks for the week, including fruits and veggies and any recipe you might want to make in advance on the weekend.

- Go through your meal plan once it's complete and make a detailed grocery list of everything you need.

- Check your fridge, freezer and pantry to see what you already have and can cross off that list.

- Go shopping and get everything you need on Friday or Saturday.

- Schedule a morning, afternoon or evening on the weekend to make whatever you need/want to prepare in advance of your week.

- Remember to check the meal plan every evening to make sure you know what's coming up the next day.

- Be flexible. Stuff happens. Always have the fixings for a couple of healthy fast food options in the pantry just in case.

## Cooking for One (or Two)

It's easy to lose motivation to keep things varied, fresh and healthy when you are cooking for only one or two people, and it can also be an expensive undertaking without planning. Here are some of my best tips for keeping your meals healthy and your budget intact when cooking for one or two:

- Meal plan! Repeat some basic ingredients each week to reduce waste. For example, have hot pasta with sauce one night, and use the leftover noodles as the basis for a pasta salad for a lunch option.

- Shop bulk but shop small. The advantage of bulk-bin shopping is you can buy small amounts of dry goods like nuts, seeds, flours and grains, allowing you to spend less and buy fresher ingredients.

- Invest in a great set of freezer-safe containers and make friends with your freezer.

- Avoid recipes with rare ingredients you won't use often.

- Make a habit of cooking on the weekend and eating those dishes all week. Make a soup or chili for lunches and roast a chicken. Freeze half of everything you make.

- Single-portion your purchases, like meat and seafood, before freezing.

- Search the internet for "healthy recipes for one," or divide recipes for two in half.

- Better yet, become a master of cooking without recipes by finding herb and spice combinations you enjoy, which allows you to always cook just enough for yourself. Stir-fries, egg dishes and salads are easily customized for one.

- Always keep on hand the ingredients for one or two healthy fast food meals such as breakfast for dinner, pita pizzas or whole grain pasta with tomato sauce and frozen edamame.

- Embrace frozen produce. Frozen veggies, fruits and berries are often as nutrient-dense as their fresh counterparts, last for ages and can be used as needed when recipes call for fresh.

- If produce is sold by weight, don't be shy about breaking it up (take a couple of bananas or a half a bunch of broccoli, for example.)

- Freeze leftover fresh herbs by blending them with olive oil in a food processor, then freezing in ice-cube trays for individually sized portions. Herbs like basil, cilantro and parsley freeze really well this way!

- Get together with some single friends and organize a "recipe swap." Everyone makes one healthy, big-batch, freezable meal and divides it into single portions. Then you all swap your extras and leave with a variety of frozen meals for the week.

- Start a cooking club with friends. One member hosts a group meal each week. Healthy and fun!

## STEP 2: KNOWING YOUR OPTIONS

Trust me, food shopping doesn't need to be a dreaded weekly chore. If you're properly organized, it can be efficient, pleasant and even downright rewarding.

There are lots of different places to buy real food. Depending on your current shopping practices and your schedule, you may decide to shop at one or more locations. How many stops you make is completely up to you — the objective is not to overwhelm you, but to empower you and make life easier, and that end goal will be achieved in different ways for different families.

The vast majority of the ingredients in my recipes and meal plans can be purchased at a conventional grocery store, so you can get away with buying all of your real food in one convenient location (with the exception of a couple harder to find ingredients that you might need to stock up on at the natural food or bulk store once every few months). That said, there may be an advantage to shopping at your local farmers' market, health food store or bulk food store, or even joining a local Community Supported Agriculture (CSA) farm share program, though it's generally less convenient to shop in more than one place. You need to weigh the pros and cons and decide what works best for you. Remember that for most people, making changes gradually will be far more effective than trying to do it all at once. Your best bet may be to start off shopping for most items at a conventional grocery store, and then slowly begin to take advantage of what the other shopping options can offer you.

For example, a nearby farmers' market will offer local produce that is very often fresher than the produce in the grocery store and, usually, also lower priced. You may also be able to get items like whole grain bread without any additives, pastured chicken and eggs (true free-range eggs come from hens that roam freely outdoors, in a pasture or woodland, where they can forage for their natural diet), grass-fed beef and even local dairy products like fresh yoghurt and cheese.

Bulk or wholesale food stores often offer many real food ingredients at a discounted price. Foods like whole grains, whole grain flours, arrowroot powder, almond milk, apple butter, dried beans and legumes, nuts and seeds, nut butters and a huge variety of spices are often available at a better price than at the grocery store.

If you're not familiar with a CSA arrangement, it's a way for the community to support local farmers by committing to purchase a share of farmed produce, meat, eggs or other real food items in advance of the farming season. This allows farmers to finance their operations, and shareholders receive a weekly basket of locally farmed foods in exchange.

Of course, the cheapest place to shop is your own backyard! If you enjoy gardening, or have been thinking about starting a garden, this is a great way to provide some of your own organic, local produce for very little money. If you're hesitant to start off with a full-scale garden, or don't have any yard space, simple deck planters are a great way to start cultivating your green thumb. Every year, in addition to my raised-bed vegetable garden, I grow a wide variety of herbs and a few tomato plants on my back deck, which costs me next to nothing. Again, remember that none of these suggestions need to happen right away (or even at all), but can be slowly incorporated into your family's life as you get better and better at planning, prepping and cooking real food.

## STEP 3: BECOMING A GROCERY-STORE NINJA

As much as I would love to avoid the conventional grocery store altogether, it's just not practical or even possible given where I live, which is probably also the case for most of you. Making the unavoidable weekly visit to the grocery store less painful involves a few tricks:

- **Make your list!** Get very good at making a precise grocery list that incorporates all of the ingredients you need for your weekly meal plan as well as items that you'll need for healthy snacks and any last minute, unplanned "fast food dinners." Start by going through the Staples List (pages 170–180) to make sure you're not running low on any of those ingredients. Then, using one of my meal plans or one you have designed for the week, review the plan and recipes very carefully, and add everything you need to make that meal plan happen. Add to that list whatever you need to keep your family well stocked in healthy snacks for the week, and then check to see that you have the ingredients for at least one of the healthy fast food dinners (page 169). Hopefully, you won't need to use them, but it's always best to prepare for even the best-laid plans falling through!

- **Organize your list for maximum efficiency and minimal frustration.** In the grocery lists that accompany the meal plans in this program, I've grouped ingredients generally by food type and the area of the grocery store where they are likely found (i.e., produce, natural food, canned goods, dairy) to make shopping easier, and recommend you do the same when you're making your own grocery list — it reduces the likelihood of having to to zigzag back and forth across the store.

- **Check your list twice!** Double-check your list to ensure you haven't left off anything critical.

- **Stick to it!** This is crucial. Did you know that seven out of every ten purchases are spontaneous? Avoid that trap by knowing exactly what you need and buying only what's on your awesome and complete list.

- **Plan for a pleasant experience!** Go to the grocery store during off-hours whenever you can, like first thing in the morning or after dinner. Eat a healthy meal or snack before you go to reduce the likelihood of spontaneous, craving-driven purchases. Combined with your ultra-organized and streamlined grocery list, this kind of planning can make the trip positively Zen!

- **Shop the perimeter but don't be afraid to go elsewhere!** You've probably heard that the healthiest food in the grocery store is found around the outside edges, which is generally true. However, you can't ignore the rest of the store. The natural food section, where many of the healthy ingredients you'll be using regularly are found, is often located more centrally. A few of the other ingredients on your list will be found in the internal aisles, such as canned tomatoes and beans, vegetable and chicken broth and dried beans and rice.

- **Shop high and low, literally.** This is a great way to cut down on your grocery bill. Did you know that the most expensive items are almost always placed at eye level, with bargains on the lower and upper shelves?

- **Buy in bulk when it makes sense.** Be aware of unit prices and take advantage of sales. The bigger the container, the lower the price per unit, generally. However if you "go big" and can't get through it all before it goes bad, is the larger size worth it? If you can freeze it, it usually makes sense to buy healthy food in bulk (or when it's on sale).

- **Buy local, in-season produce.** It is almost always cheaper than imported, non-seasonal produce. A trip to your local farmers' market will often get you even better deals. For veggies and fruits that are not locally grown in the winter, the frozen version is often a great way to eat healthily and inexpensively.

- **Buy organic when you can, but don't pay for organic if you can't afford it.** If you are concerned about pesticides, you can use the Dirty Dozen and Clean Fifteen, a list you can download for free from me at **www.formaclorimerbooks.ca/realfood/dirtydozen.pdf** that identifies the twelve most contaminated fruits and veggies, as a guide for what to buy organic.

- **Buy less meat.** Meat is *really* expensive, especially the good quality stuff. Cut back on your family's meat intake by incorporating vegetarian protein. My meal plans contain lots of tasty vegetarian main meals, but if you're doing your own meal planning, try to incorporate at least two vegetarian meals a week. Beans and tofu are *cheap*, so this change alone can help you save big.

- **Consider buying dried beans and peas over canned.** Dried beans are very cheap and cooking them is actually quite easy. On top of saving money, by using dried beans you can eliminate sodium, avoid the BPA in can liners and increase the digestibility of the beans through proper soaking and cooking methods. For soaking and easy cooking instructions, download a free Bean Guide from me at **www.formaclorimerbooks.ca/realfood/beanguide.pdf**.

- **Do a pre-checkout cart check.** Before you check out, check out your cart. Is most of what's in there real food, with only one ingredient? Can you see a rainbow of colour, or are you lacking variety? Have you got at least one dark, leafy green veggie in there, such as spinach, kale, collards or chard? Are there any items you spontaneously added to your cart that are not as healthy and that you can do without? Dump them!

## STEP 4: ESSENTIAL KITCHEN NINJA TOOLS

Cooking is so much more pleasant when you have a few efficient tools on hand to make your life easier. I don't believe you need a lot of fancy stuff to cook great food, but the few gadgets I do use are well worth the investment. You can build your kitchen tool box slowly; there is no need to buy all of these items up front.

- **Food processor:** This is the only bigger ticket item on my list, but it is so helpful, it will pay for itself in saved time in the first month alone and you'll wonder why it took you so long to get one. Check around, you may just have a family member who has one that's gathering dust. Look for a large bowl (eleven or more cups), otherwise you'll likely be upgrading in a year. You can also often get these on sale and should be able to find a good quality food processor for under $200.

- **Citrus squeezer:** This little press squeezes citrus with no effort, so nothing goes to waste. So much easier to use than an old-fashioned hand juicer! You can find one for under $15 at your local kitchen store.

- **Garlic press:** I've heard many a fancy-pants gourmet type diss the humble garlic press, but I will never give mine up in exchange for peeling and chopping cloves by hand. It's time-consuming and, let's face it, stinky. A press allows you to crush the unpeeled clove, extracting the garlic quickly. A must-have when you love garlic like I do, a good garlic press will cost around $20 and last for ages.

- **Very fine grater (or "microplane"):** This very fine, flat grater grates fresh or frozen ginger, lemon or lime rind and Parmesan or Asiago like a dream, so I never use my larger box grater for any of these foods. Cleanup is way easier with a flat fine grater. This will set you back only about $15.

- **Good chef's knife:** You don't really need a full set of good quality knives, although I do recommend it if you've got the budget for it. If not, just invest in one good quality chef's knife (the big one), which most kitchen stores sell separately. This is a more expensive purchase, but if it's taken care of, it will last a lifetime. Wait until there's a sale, or shop online, and you can pick a decent one up for around $100.

- **Storage containers, in various sizes, for freezing:** Unless you've got loads of time on your hands, chances are a big part of your ability to stay on track will depend on batch cooking and freezing. In order to make that work, you obviously need good quality freezer-safe containers. I recommend you buy containers suited for both individual portions and family-sized meals. You have lots of options. Ovenproof glass containers with plastic lids, Mason jars, BPA-free plastic containers and freezer bags are all useful. If you're freezing in Mason jars, remember to leave a little space at the top to allow for expansion, otherwise you'll have one big mess on your hands!

- **A set of good quality containers for packed lunches and snacks:** If you work or spend most days outside of your home, you'll also need to pack your lunch and snacks daily in order to stay on track with your food, so you'll want some practical, portable food containers. A small, good quality Thermos is a great way to transport hot soups and stews. An insulated lunch bag with a gel ice pack will help keep food chilled and fresh. There are lots of nifty containers out there these days that can make packing your lunch more pleasant, including beverage containers with a frozen core to keep smoothies cold and salad containers with different compartments to keep ingredients crispy until lunchtime.

## STEP 5: BECOMING A KITCHEN NINJA

### Preparation is Key!

These basic cooking strategies and kitchen habits will make your life so much easier if you can just get them down to a science. First, start to consistently look at what's happening the next day in terms of your meal plan, and make sure you are ready to execute that. This might mean doing some prep work in advance, such as making some brown rice, peeling and chopping veggies for a recipe or pre-cooking lentils or beans. You'll see that at the beginning of each weekly meal plan I've identified some advance prep work that will allow you to stay on plan for the rest of the week. I highly recommend you get that done every weekend along with hard-boiling a half a dozen eggs and making some hummus or salad dressing if you've run out.

### Batch Cooking and Doubling Up

I also recommend that, whenever you're making a recipe, you consider making double and freezing half. This is one of the most useful habits you can get into, because you'll quickly build up a collection of frozen meals that you can use on busy weeknights. Most of the recipes in this cookbook freeze well. Generally speaking, recipes containing cooked pasta or with a milk or cream base don't freeze as well, in that their consistency may change slightly upon defrosting and reheating. Other than that, most recipes are safe to freeze for at least three months (longer if they're vegetarian). In the meal plans I sometimes specifically advise you to make extra and freeze a portion — for example, it's just as easy to roast two chickens as one, and roasting two will give you sandwich meat and toppings for your salad for the rest of the week, so that just makes sense.

So set aside two to three hours on Sundays, crank up the tunes and get your kitchen groove on! Better yet, invite a friend over and batch cook together, sharing the spoils and stocking two freezers in the process. Your weekdays will be immeasurably more pleasant if you get into this weekend routine.

### Freeze It, Don't Waste It!

Another time and money saver in the kitchen is freezing ingredients before they go bad and need to be composted. You'll be amazed to know some of the following real food items you can freeze to save money and avoid waste.

**Fresh herbs:** I often use fresh herbs in my recipes, because they add amazing flavour, but it's difficult to use up an entire bunch of parsley or cilantro before it starts to wilt. You can keep your herbs fresh for longer by placing them upright in some water, but you can also simply combine them with a little bit of olive oil in the food processor and then freeze that mixture in tablespoon-sized portions on a tray covered in wax paper or parchment. Once they're frozen, just pop them off the sheet and into a Baggie and label it. The next time you need a tablespoon of cilantro or parsley you can save money by using what you've got in the freezer instead of buying another fresh bunch.

**Grated lemon and lime rind:** You can also freeze lemon and lime rind, so it's a great idea to always zest your citrus before you juice it, even if the recipe doesn't call for the rind as well. Keep a couple of containers in your freezer for lemon and lime rind and this trick will save you time and money.

**Ginger root:** Rarely will you buy fresh ginger and be able to use it all before it starts to rot. When I buy fresh ginger root, I peel the skin back and grate whatever I need for the recipe and then wrap the rest in plastic wrap and store it in a freezer Baggie. The next time I need ginger, I just peel the skin back with a knife and grate it frozen, usually doubling the amount the recipe calls for (frozen ginger root has the consistency of shaved ice and you'll need more of it than you would if you were grating it fresh).

**Cooked brown rice:** Brown rice freezes well, so make double and freeze it in 1/2 cup portions to grab and take with soup or chili for a healthy lunch.

**Hummus:** Freeze hummus in an ice-cube tray for perfect portions you can pop into your lunch bag frozen (it will defrost by lunchtime).

**Pesto:** Another great use for fresh herbs is to whip them up into a quick pesto. Combine herbs (basil, parsley or cilantro work well) with olive oil, some nuts or seeds (pine nuts, walnuts and pumpkin seeds are my favourites), a cup or two of spinach or kale, fresh garlic and sea salt and purée until smooth in a food processor. I like to freeze pesto in an ice-cube tray for convenience; a thawed cube will dress roasted or grilled veggies, coat a big bowl of pasta, marinate chicken or fish, top a homemade pizza and make a great base for a salad dressing.

**Leftover tomato paste:** How many times have you used a couple tablespoons of tomato paste in a recipe and thrown the rest out? Never again! Scoop leftover tomato paste into a container and freeze, labelling with the amount.

**Leftover coconut milk:** Another often-wasted ingredient, there's nothing worse than needing only half a can and watching the rest go to waste. Freeze it!

**Cherry tomatoes:** Throw cherry tomatoes into a freezer Baggie or container and they can be used later in soups, sauces and stews.

**Chickpeas and beans:** It makes sense to start cooking your beans from dried — it costs about a sixth of the price of canned and is usually a healthier choice. I cook mine about once every six weeks, making large batches of two or three types of bean and then letting them cool after rinsing. I freeze the cooked beans in freezer bags in 1 1/2 cup portions — about the equivalent of a typical 14 oz can of beans. When a recipe calls for a can of beans, I just grab a bag from my freezer.

**Tofu:** This is a great tip for those who are cooking for one, as a block of tofu will feed four to five people. Cut what you need from the tofu block, cut the rest into cubes, then freeze on a tray or plate, transferring cubes to a container once frozen. When you are ready to use the frozen tofu, thaw on the counter and use as if it was fresh.

## STEP 6: BECOMING A HEALTHY FAST FOOD NINJA

Here are my five "Old Faithfuls": the quick and healthy last-minute meals I default to on rushed evenings to save my family and me from ordering in or eating out. You probably have a couple of your own, so add them to this list and tape it to the inside of a cupboard door, then use it to gather your thoughts and save the day when chaos hits.

- **Breakfast for dinner:** Scrambled eggs, raw fruit and veggies, whole grain toast with peanut or almond butter.

- **Whole grain pasta and natural spaghetti sauce (jarred):** Boil noodles, heat up sauce and add a protein (canned beans, frozen edamame, pre-cooked chicken or cubed tofu). You can also add chopped spinach to the sauce to "pump it up" while it's heating on the stove.

- **Pita pizzas:** Whole grain pitas topped with jarred spaghetti sauce, chopped veggies and grated cheese, then baked at 375°F for 10 to 15 minutes. Serve with an easy side salad or raw veggies.

- **The big salad (serves one):** 2 cups salad greens, 1 cup chopped raw veggies, 1/3 to 1/2 cup protein of choice (beans, chickpeas, cooked chicken or shrimp), 1 to 2 tbsp healthy dressing, 1 to 2 tsp pumpkin or sunflower seeds or slivered almonds.

- **Super-fast stir-fry:** In large pan, melt 1 tbsp of coconut oil. Add 4 to 6 cups shredded and/or chopped veggies of choice (carrots, cabbage, beets, etc.) and 1 to 2 crushed garlic cloves. Sauté until soft. Toss in some pre-cooked chicken, cubed tofu or beans and heat through. Add a quick sauce (see Stir It Up!, page 139, for two sauce options) or just stir in a little low-sodium soy sauce and a splash of sesame oil. Serve over defrosted and reheated pre-cooked brown rice.

# CHAPTER 19

# Pantry, Fridge and Freezer Staples List

| Almond butter | This is a great alternative to peanut butter that is acceptable during the Cleanstart week of the program, and can be substituted for peanut butter in just about any recipe. (Look for a natural version made with just almonds and no added sugars.) | Natural food section of conventional grocery store<br><br>Natural food store<br><br>Bulk store |
|---|---|---|
| Almond milk (unsweetened) | Almond milk is my dairy alternative of choice, so I use that in my recipes in the place of milk. My whole family prefers its taste and consistency to other alternatives. That said, feel free to use unsweetened soy or rice milk in my recipes if you are nut-free or just prefer it. Those will work as well. | Natural food section of conventional grocery store (cooler or shelf, depending on packaging)<br><br>Natural food store |
| Almonds (raw) | Almonds make a perfect protein and healthy fat-based portable snack and are a great staple to always have on hand. Carry a small container in your bag and keep the rest in the fridge. | Bulk section of conventional grocery store<br><br>Natural food store<br><br>Bulk store |

| | | |
|---|---|---|
| Apple butter | This is a wonderful, naturally sweet alternative to jam made with apples. (Look for one with no added sugars.) It freezes well, so consider freezing half to extend its life. | Natural food section of conventional grocery store<br><br>Natural food store<br><br>Bulk store |
| Apple cider vinegar | This healthy vinegar has been used in natural health remedies for centuries. Always look for a brand that is "with mother" to ensure the nutritious bits haven't been filtered out. The bottle will clearly state this on the label. | Vinegar/oils section or natural food section of conventional grocery store<br><br>Natural food store |
| Applesauce (unsweetened) | I use unsweetened applesauce in many of my basic baking recipes to add natural sweetness and moisture. I always have a jar in my pantry or fridge. | Condiment or natural food section of conventional grocery store |
| Arrowroot powder or flour | A natural thickener made from the arrowroot plant, this can replace cornstarch (which is generally made from GM corn) or gluten-containing flours as a thickener. | Natural food store<br><br>Bulk store |
| Baking powder (aluminum-free) | Ingested aluminum has been linked to health issues, so why take the chance? Use aluminum-free baking powder. | Natural food section of conventional grocery store<br><br>Natural food store<br><br>Bulk store |
| Balsamic vinegar | This is a pantry essential when you make your own salad dressings. In fact, some of the better quality balsamics are so delicious they make a great dressing drizzled solo on fresh veggies. | Vinegar/oils section of conventional grocery store |

| | | |
|---|---|---|
| Brown rice | This gluten-free whole grain will become a staple in your real food diet. It makes a good base for a chili or stir-fry or as a side dish with any meal. There are many varieties to choose from — personally I prefer short-grain or brown basmati rice because of their sweet, nutty flavours. | Rice and pasta section or natural food section of conventional grocery store<br><br>Bulk store |
| Brown rice pasta | A gluten-free pasta made from whole grain rice. Cook it, rinse it well, then reheat under hot water for best results. | Natural food section of conventional grocery store<br><br>Bulk store |
| Brown rice cakes | I always have these on hand for emergency snack attacks. Spread with almond butter and apple butter, or top with hummus and avocado. | Natural food section of conventional grocery store<br><br>Natural food store |
| Chickpeas (canned or dried) | The main ingredient in hummus, I also use chickpeas in many main dishes so you'll always want to have a few cans on hand (or cook a big batch from dried and freeze the beans in can-sized portions of 1 1/2 cups. For instructions, download my Bean Guide for free at **www.formaclorimerbooks.ca/ realfood/beanguide.pdf**). If using canned, look for BPA-free cans to avoid this known endocrine disruptor commonly used in can linings. | Natural food section (for BPA-free cans) or soup section (for dried) of conventional grocery store<br><br>Natural food store<br><br>Bulk store for dried beans |
| Coconut (unsweetened, shredded) | I use unsweetened shredded coconut for sweetness and flavour in recipes and recommend you have it on hand. | Baking section of conventional grocery store<br><br>Natural food section of conventional grocery store (for organic version)<br><br>Bulk store |

| Coconut milk | Available in a can or carton, this makes a great dairy alternative in creamy soups and curries. You can choose a lower-fat version to reduce calories and also look for lower-sugar content, which varies between brands. | Natural food or international food section of conventional grocery store (look in the cooler for cartons and on the shelf for cans) |
|---|---|---|
| Coconut oil | A stable fat, coconut oil is fantastic for cooking at a high temperature, as it doesn't break down or lose its healthy properties. The virgin oil will have a sweet, slightly "coconutty" flavour, whereas, non-virgin has no odour or flavour. Use it for cooking and as a replacement for vegetable or canola oil in baking (melt it first!). Note that it's solid at room temperature, and comes in a jar not a bottle. | Natural food section of conventional grocery store<br><br>Natural food store |
| Dates (dried) | Dates are an essential ingredient in many of my dessert and treat recipes as their natural sweetness allows me to use less maple syrup or other sweetener. I prefer medjool dates, because they tend to be moister and easier to chop and use. If your dates are dry, you can usually reconstitute them by soaking them in a bowl of hot water for a few minutes. | Produce section of conventional grocery store for medjool dates<br><br>Baking aisle of conventional grocery store for other packaged dried dates<br><br>Bulk store |
| Dijon mustard (creamy, not grainy) | Dijon mustard adds a zip to dressings and savoury recipes. I always have a jar of the creamy version in my fridge. | Condiments section of conventional grocery store<br><br>Natural food section of conventional grocery store for organic version |

| | | |
|---|---|---|
| Edamame | Edamame is the Japanese name for young soybeans. Buy these green beans frozen (shelled or unshelled) then defrost and heat for a quick source of complete protein. | Natural foods section (freezer) of conventional grocery store |
| Eggs | Eggs make a satisfying protein-rich snack. You'll see I use them often in meal-plan breakfasts and main meal recipes so you'll always want to have some on hand. If possible, buy eggs from pastured hens. | Conventional grocery store (cooler)<br><br>Natural food store (cooler)<br><br>Farmers' market |
| Egg whites (liquid) | Pure liquid egg whites are a great way to add protein without adding too many calories (look for one ingredient only: "liquid egg whites"). Don't skip the yolk, though, that's where the bulk of the nutrition is. I recommend 1 egg and 1/4 cup of egg whites for breakfast to keep you going longer. | Conventional grocery store (cooler section, by the whole eggs) |
| Flax oil | Derived from flax, this oil is a terrific source of healthy, anti-inflammatory omega-3. A delicate fat, it should be refrigerated and never heated. Great in cold salad dressings or smoothies. | Natural food section (cooler) of conventional grocery store<br><br>Natural food store |
| Garlic | Garlic is one of my favourite savoury ingredients, so you'll want to always have it on hand if you're using my recipes. It adds terrific flavour and depth to even simple recipes. Plus it's naturally antibacterial and supportive of immune health. | Produce section of conventional grocery store<br><br>Farmers' market |
| Ground flaxseed or flax meal | Flaxseed is a good source of omega-3, but its nutrients are best absorbed when ground. Buy flaxseed and grind it yourself or just buy the pre-ground meal. Store it in the fridge. | Natural food section of conventional grocery store<br><br>Natural food store<br><br>Bulk store |

| | | |
|---|---|---|
| Honey | Honey is my sweetener of choice for most dressings. Buy local honey if you can find it. | Conventional grocery store<br><br>Natural food store |
| Lentils, green and red (dried) | Lentils are a cheap source of quality protein and an easy legume to cook with because they don't require any presoaking. After a quick scan for damaged beans and foreign bits like grains or small pebbles, give the lentils a rinse and cook them 18 to 20 minutes, either on their own or in a soup or stew. | Soup/bean section or natural food section of conventional grocery store<br><br>Natural food store<br><br>Bulk store |
| Low-sodium soy sauce or tamari | Chinese soy sauce often contains wheat as well as soy, while the Japanese version, tamari, is usually wheat- and gluten-free. My favourite brand is Bragg soy seasoning (or Bragg Liquid Aminos) as it's wheat-free, made from non-GMO soy and has a lovely, light flavour. | Natural food section of conventional grocery store<br><br>Natural food store |
| Maple syrup | A little goes a long way with this natural sweetener. You will use it on oatmeal and in recipes, so it's a good condiment to always have on hand. Always buy the real thing; pancake syrups are full of artificial ingredients and refined sugar. | Conventional grocery store<br><br>Natural food store<br><br>Bulk store |
| Nutritional (or vegetarian) yeast or yeast flakes | Normally fortified with vitamin B12, this is a deactivated yellow, flaked yeast that imparts a cheesy, tangy flavour to dairy-free dishes. | Natural food section of conventional grocery store<br><br>Natural food store |

| | | |
|---|---|---|
| Oats (plain, unsweetened)<br><br>You will need to stock 3 types: Slow-cook rolled oats, which take more than 5 minutes to cook and work better in most baking recipes. If the label says they cook in less than 5 minutes, they are quick oats; quick (or instant) oats, which cook in 5 minutes or less and can be microwaved; and steel-cut oats, which take about 20 minutes to cook on the stove. | Oats are a really useful staple in a real food pantry because they can be used in so many contexts: cooked in hot water for a quick breakfast, used in baked goods, ground to replace bread crumbs in a veggie burger or meatloaf or soaked overnight with milk and fruit for a cold morning muesli. Have all three types on hand; they'll all come in handy when you're following this program. | Baking section (for slow-cook rolled oats) and cereal section (for quick/instant and steel-cut oats) of conventional grocery store<br><br>Natural food section of conventional grocery store or natural food store (for organic versions)<br><br>Bulk store |
| Olive oil | This is my standard healthy oil for cooking at a low to medium temperature, but not at a high heat. It also makes a great base for homemade dressings. Don't cheap out on this; it's worth spending a little more for better quality and taste. | Natural food section and oil/vinegar section of conventional grocery store<br><br>Natural food store |

| | | |
|---|---|---|
| Plain Greek yoghurt | A thick yoghurt that is high in protein and a source of healthy probiotics, this makes a great base for dips and sauces or more generally as a replacement for sour cream. Look for 18 to 20 g of protein per serving and no added sugars. In a pinch, a plain non-Greek variety will usually work in my recipes too. | Dairy cooler of conventional grocery store |
| Popcorn | Best real food snack ever! Pop kernels in a little coconut oil and sprinkle with nutritional yeast and/or sea salt to stop a crunchy, salty craving in its tracks. I always have some on hand. | Snack aisle, bulk area or natural food section of conventional grocery store<br><br>Bulk store |
| Quinoa | Another gluten-free whole grain, this is technically a seed. It cooks in 20 minutes or less and has a mild taste that's perfect as a base for almost any flavour combination. Rinse in a fine mesh strainer before cooking to remove any traces of the bitter coating that is often found on quinoa. | Rice and pasta section or natural food section of conventional grocery store<br><br>Bulk store |
| Red wine vinegar | This is another vinegar that's great in salad dressings and good to have in your cupboard for a last-minute vinaigrette. | Oil/vinegar section of conventional grocery store<br><br>Natural food section of conventional grocery store (organic version) |
| Sea salt | I like to keep a grinder for coarse sea salt (for use as a garnish) and a jar of finer-ground sea salt (for use in recipes) in my kitchen. I prefer the flavour of sea salt, and it also contains important trace minerals that have been stripped from the average processed table salt. | Baking/spice section or natural food section of conventional grocery store |

| Seeds | Raw seeds make a great addition to salads and oatmeal — they add crunch, flavour and healthy fat. I recommend always having some pumpkin or sunflower seeds in your fridge. | Bulk section or natural food section (for organic versions) of conventional grocery store<br><br>Natural food store<br><br>Bulk store |
|---|---|---|
| Spelt flour | A grain in the wheat family, spelt is lower in gluten and easier to digest for many than conventional wheat. It's easy to substitute into basic baking recipes like pancakes, pizza dough and tortillas. | Natural food section of conventional grocery store (for organic versions)<br><br>Natural food store<br><br>Bulk store |
| Spices, dried | A well-stocked spice drawer is a must in a real food kitchen. While my recipes often call for fresh herbs and occasionally for a less-common dried spice, I use a core group of dried spices and recommend you have these on hand:<br><br>Allspice<br>Basil<br>Black pepper (ground)<br>Cayenne pepper<br>Chili powder<br>Cilantro<br>Cinnamon (ground)<br>Cloves (ground)<br>Coriander (ground)<br>Cumin (ground)<br>Curry powder<br>Crushed red pepper (red pepper flakes)<br>Dill<br>Ginger (ground)<br>Nutmeg (ground)<br>Oregano<br>Paprika<br>Rosemary<br>Sage<br>Smoked Paprika<br>Thyme<br>Turmeric | Spice aisle of conventional grocery store<br><br>Natural food section of conventional grocery store (for organic versions)<br><br>Natural food store (for organic versions)<br><br>Bulk store |

| | | |
|---|---|---|
| Stevia | A natural sweetener derived from the stevia plant, this is available in liquid or powder form and is acceptable to use during the Cleanstart week of my program. It's very sweet-tasting, so go easy. Remember that sweetness in any form feeds sugar cravings! | Natural food section or baking section of conventional grocery store<br><br>Natural food store |
| Tahini (or, as it is sometimes called, Tahina or Tahineh) | Tahini is a ground sesame seed paste that is a source of healthy fat and provides amazing flavour to salad dressings and sauces. | International food section or natural food section of conventional grocery store<br><br>Natural food store<br><br>Bulk store |
| Toasted sesame oil | Just a small amount of this very flavourful oil goes a long, long way. It makes a wonderful addition to stir-fries and dressings. Untoasted plain sesame oil is sometimes easier to find and substitutes well. | Natural food or Asian food section of conventional grocery store<br><br>Natural food store<br><br>Asian grocery store |
| Tofu (firm or soft) | Made from soybeans, tofu is an inexpensive, complete protein. As most conventional soybeans have been genetically modified, always choose organic tofu or look for non-GMO soybeans in the ingredient list. Once opened, cover remaining tofu with water and store in fridge for 3 to 5 days, changing water daily, or wrap well and freeze. Be sure to check the specific type of tofu called for in a recipe — firm tofu and extra-soft tofu have very different consistencies and are generally not interchangeable. | Natural food section of conventional grocery store (cooler or shelf, depending on packaging)<br><br>Natural food store |

| Tomatoes, diced, crushed and whole (canned or jarred) | Canned (or jarred) tomatoes form the basis of many of my recipes so keep your pantry stocked. I always have in my pantry a couple of cans of each type: diced, crushed and whole. | Canned vegetable area or natural food section (for organic versions) of conventional grocery store |
|---|---|---|
| Vanilla extract (real, not artificial) | Real vanilla extract adds sweetness to breakfasts and baked goods and is a staple in my kitchen. | Baking aisle or natural food section of conventional grocery store. Natural food store |
| Vegetable broth (low-sodium) | Whenever my favourite vegetable broth goes on sale, I stock up. The basis for most of my soups and stews, a few cartons are a pantry staple. If you're not vegetarian, you can always use low-sodium chicken broth. | Natural food section or soup section of conventional grocery store Natural food store |
| White wine vinegar | A tasty, basic vinegar, this gets used in my dressings and sauces regularly to add a little tang. | Vinegar/oils section of conventional grocery store |
| Whole wheat flour (organic or all-natural) | Buy organic — the conventional whole wheat flours usually have a bunch of additives. | Natural food section of conventional grocery store Natural food store |
| Yellow prepared mustard | Yellow mustard adds zip to recipes. Look for one without artificial colour in the natural food section. | Condiments section or natural food section (for organic, no-colour-added version) of conventional grocery store |

# CHAPTER 20

## Family Matters

If you're hoping to improve your family's food in addition to taking up the challenge of changing your personal diet for the better, bravo! You care enough about what your kids are eating to work at improving it, and you have lots of great reasons to do so. Everything in previous chapters about why eating real food matters to you applies equally to your kids. They, too, feel a million times better with balanced blood sugar and an overflowing vitamin and mineral bank account!

I'm no stranger to the challenges involved in getting kids to eat less processed food and more fruits and vegetables. I've helped many families change the "food dynamic" at their dinner table. I'm also raising two of my own small people, each with their own quirks and food preferences that have lead to our own share of family food challenges.

Raising healthy eaters is worth the work you'll put in, and it *can* be done, even in families with the pickiest eaters. The effective, kid-tested strategies in this chapter will get your children (and spouse) excited about making healthy changes to your family's food, and will get them involved in and contributing to planning, prepping and cooking. Not only will my strategies lighten your load, they will give your kids the skills they need to leave your home and be healthy eaters for life. Two birds. One stone.

Healthy food needs to taste good *and* be fun — this core belief underpins all of my strategies. If your table, like so many of the families I've worked with, has become a battleground, get ready to flip the switch by completely eliminating any and all negativity surrounding food. Just like everything else, it's about slow, steady change, consistency and positive reinforcement — and I'm about to lay it out for you, step by step.

## MAKING CHANGE

How do you get started? First, have a private discussion as parents to make sure you're clear about what you want to accomplish. Are you hoping to get your family to an 80/20 balance? Would you like to waste less food or eat out less often? Do you have a child who needs to eat more vegetables or broaden his palate? Maybe you'd just like to get to a place where everyone sits down and eats the same healthy meal with no complaining.

Second, get on the same page when it comes to the language and parenting approach you are going to use. Consistency is key; this process will be a whole lot smoother if you can rely on each other as backup. Staying calm and positive is also a must — when you feel your blood pressure rising, being able to rely on someone else to calmly take the reins is so helpful!

Once you've arrived at a consensus and identified some priorities, it's time for a family meeting. This is when you really need to sell this thing, with unbridled, (bordering on ridiculous) positivity and excitement. And I mean "This is going to be the most fun thing *ever*" kind of positivity. Don't single out any one member of your family, like a particularly picky eater, as being the "problem." Instead, take the blame as parents for not focusing the way you should have on making sure everybody's getting the support they need to eat and enjoy lots of healthy food. Trust me, kids love it when parents admit they've made a mistake, so this is a really great place to start. Singling out one picky eater in your family is just going to provide that child with more attention, which often adds fuel to the fire.

Start out with everybody on an even playing field, working together as a family unit to improve your food and get healthy. Call it "Project Healthy Family," and talk about what you would all like to see in terms of positive changes. It helps to identify one unique weakness for each member of your family to work on, even the parents and better eaters. Maybe you usually buy your lunch instead of packing it, so that's what you're going to work on, and Dad just doesn't eat enough salad, so he's going to try to pack a salad every day. In all likelihood, your kids aren't eating the minimum recommended five servings of fruits and veggies a day, so that's a great place for them to start. Or maybe you have some veggie lovers who tend to eat the same things over and over again, so they need to focus on getting more variety. The key is to make sure everyone is working on something specific, so there's an opportunity for everyone to succeed.

Next, make everyone accountable, but in a fun way! Challenges are best met with a little healthy competition and (non-food) rewards. Start by having each family member take my "High-Five Pledge," promising to try to eat five or more servings of fruits and veggies a day (**www.formaclorimerbooks.ca/realfood/highfive.pdf**). While not all families need them (just the idea of a fun family project is enough to motivate change in some kids), I love a good reward chart (download my template at **www.formaclorimerbooks.ca/realfood/reward.pdf**). There's nothing more motivating than a fridge with a reward chart for every family member, including Mom and Dad. You're not rewarding *eating* but healthy, positive behaviours, with the goal of developing permanent habits. When your husband eats salad, you're rewarding the effort and planning involved in choosing, making and eating a home-packed lunch. When a picky eater who throws a nightly tantrum at the family table tries a new food without making a fuss, you're rewarding a job well done. After a week (or less, you decide) of each family member "doing their job," there's a reward earned. The trick is to choose a reward that they *really* want — all kids have a currency, whether it's time alone with a parent, an extra story at bedtime, a trip to the park, a new book or a dollar-store toy. It doesn't have to be expensive, and in my experience, the most effective rewards aren't material. Kids crave affection, praise and responsibility. Your enthusiasm, positive reinforcement and efforts to involve your children in family food will all go a long way when it comes to effecting change.

Post the charts and get going! Make sure before you start that your children clearly know what's expected of them, whether it's taking one bite of a new food without making a fuss, eating three veggies and two fruits a day, assembling a salad before dinner or setting and clearing the table. Remind them of the specifics of their "job" and exactly what they can expect when they accomplish it (i.e., a sticker on the chart, and after a week of stickers, an earned reward). Set them up for success whenever you can — the objective is always for you to have an opportunity to praise. Keep it simple in the beginning to make success more likely, and then go completely bananas with praise when they "do their job." You want them to gain confidence in the system — both what's expected and how that behaviour will be received. Again, consistency and positivity are key.

Once you've established a pattern and your table has become a calmer, more positive space, you can build slowly on your successes. If your child has been eating three servings of veggies a day for a month or so, up the challenge to four a day, or start working on variety by incorporating a weekly "eat the rainbow" challenge. If your picky eater is consistently trying a bite of new foods without a fuss, tell them they rock and are definitely ready for a job promotion to two bites without a fuss. Just like with all other behaviour, once they're confident that they can rely on the system (including that expectations won't change without fair warning, and that they'll receive a consistent, positive response when they do what's expected), you'll eventually find rewards are no longer necessary because good habits are now in place, and everyone's enjoying the reduced stress and pressure around family food.

## GETTING YOUR KIDS IN THE KITCHEN

While you're working on individual challenges, you can start getting your whole family involved in food-related tasks (some of which can also be incorporated into the reward system), such as setting and clearing the table, washing and peeling produce, weeding the garden, keeping the grocery list current, putting groceries away, meal planning and cooking. Obviously, you'll need to keep tasks simpler for younger children, building complexity and responsibility with age.

For many kids, dinner magically "appears" on the table, lunch just finds its way into their backpack, the fridge is perpetually stocked and the dishes do themselves. When we're really busy, it's often easier to just do things ourselves. We need to make a conscious effort to involve our kids in the kitchen, because if we don't teach them the basic skills they need to choose and prepare healthy food, who will? Chances are, without these skills, they'll slip into a processed, convenient diet when they leave home, because that's what's out there for them. On the other hand, if we teach them to meal plan, shop on a budget and cook and enjoy delicious, simple, healthy food, they'll be set for life.

We're raising our kids in a world where almost everything is available premade, pre-cooked, or pre-prepared, and sadly, that food is largely responsible for rising rates of childhood obesity and type 2 diabetes. Part of raising healthy eaters means giving kids at least the basic skills they need to cook and the education on why it's so important to eat real food. If we can instill a little joy and love of cooking in the process, even better!

Get your children in the kitchen early, so it becomes a part of their daily life and your household routine. If weeknights are crazy, find some time on the weekend for the more involved tasks. Here's a list of some simple things your kids can do, even at a young age:

- **Wash and peel veggies:** Use a dull peeler; teach them to peel away from their gripping hand.

- **Strip stems and spin leafy greens:** Teach them how to remove the stems from greens like kale or chard. Invest in a basic salad spinner and they can wash and spin the greens, too. If it's a kale salad you're making, let them get their hands in there and massage the dressing into the kale leaves – it's a messy job they'll love!

- **Wash the dishes:** Even the little ones can do this. Start them with unbreakable items and slowly move them up to glassware and heavier items as they get older. Mine are eleven and wash everything now except the sharp knives.

- **Set and clear the table:** This one is such a selfish lifesaver for me and has been on the chore list since my children could carry plates. They now set for all family dinners and even fancy occasions.

- **Measure:** Teach them early how to read measuring spoons and cups, level flour, pack a cup, add a pinch, et cetera.

- **Empty the dishwasher:** Yes, your children should know where everything goes! I divide the dishwasher up between sections and we rotate through them. Even the youngest child can sort basic cutlery into the drawer.

- **Grate:** As long as we supervise younger children, there is no reason why kids can't grate cheese, lemon rind, carrots, zucchini, et cetera, using a box grater.

- **Mix, whisk and stir:** Teach them the basics — always hold the bowl with one hand while stirring with the other, add flour gradually, et cetera.

- **Design a menu:** Give them the opportunity to plan a healthy meal, and you'll be amazed at how much more involved they'll want to be in its preparation. Set healthy boundaries (i.e., dinner must contain two veggies, a protein, some healthy fat) and let them create away within those. They can then make a grocery list, find what they need with you at the store, come home, prepare the meal and even serve it in style!

- **Follow a recipe:** Start with basic, no-cook recipes like toast, smoothies or sandwiches and gradually add recipes with more steps, like hard-boiled eggs, oatmeal, basic baking and stovetop cooking. Get a recipe binder going for each child, with the recipes they have mastered and the ones they want to try, their notes on how they liked it and what they might change next time. You will be absolutely amazed at where this leads — massive amounts of confidence, creativity and pride in the kitchen.

## TABLE TALK

Don't underestimate the power of table talk — the language you use to describe your family's food and habits is so powerful. If you label your child a "picky eater," you're likely setting up a self-fulfilling prophecy. On the other hand, using positive language and requiring the same of your kids allows for progress and makes the table so much more pleasant for everyone. Instead of "I don't like broccoli," teach them to say, "I don't like broccoli yet." Instead of "This is yucky" or "I hate this," teach them to say, "It's not my favourite," and you do the same when describing their food preferences. This is so much more pleasant than crying and gagging, and kids really only need to be given acceptable language and then praised a couple of times for using it before they start to establish better habits.

My goal for each family I work with is to get them to a place where everyone sits down at the table and eats the same healthy meal without making a fuss. Doesn't that sound lovely? If you're thinking "not in my lifetime," you're not alone, but you *can* get there. Kids lack empathy when it comes to the work that's involved in putting healthy food on the table. (Most of us are so busy we've gotten into the habit of just doing it all ourselves for reasons of efficiency, so they come by their lack of empathy honestly.) It's up to us to make sure they understand the effort and time that goes into every healthy meal we serve as parents, and to set limits on the behaviour we'll allow in response to it — and it's not as hard as you might think.

A mom I worked with shared this story with me, and I've used it time and time again with other parents as a teaching tool. Like many children, her young daughter had been allowed to develop the habit of creating a gigantic fuss, including fake gagging and tears, any time something that was not her favourite was served. The family table had become an unpleasant place for everyone and this mom was at her wits' end.

After a heart-to-heart session with me, she sat her daughter down and said, "The way you behave at the table is no longer acceptable. I don't think you understand how it makes me feel when you tell me you hate what I made for dinner and start to gag, so let me try to explain it to you. You know all those drawings you bring home from school that I put up on the fridge? Well, how would you feel if one day you brought me a drawing you were proud of, and asked me what I thought, and I said, 'Actually, I really don't like this one. I don't think it's very good at all. I'm not going to put it on the fridge'? I bet you'd feel sad and rotten, and it would really hurt your feelings, because you'd worked hard on that picture and were really proud of it. Well, that's exactly how I feel when you tell me you hate the food I make or pretend you're going to throw up after you eat it. I'm busy, and it takes a lot of time and love to put healthy food on the table, so when you make a fuss it makes me feel sad and rotten, too."

Guess what? She gave her child the language to express herself without being hurtful ("It's not my favourite" or "I don't like it yet"), and her child gladly started using it. Not surprisingly, her child also started "liking" a lot more things, knowing she'd been hurting her mom's feelings, but more important, also started understanding the power she had to make her mom feel great.

I strongly believe it's our job to teach our kids about the basics of nutrition and the food system. Sure, they get a little education at school, but unfortunately most of what they know, they've learned through the media, which is largely influenced by the food industry itself. Do your kids know where their food comes from? In our modern-day, convenience-based commercialized food world, how many kids know the difference between a whole and processed food? How many have visited a working farm or grown food from seed? How many know how to read a basic food label or understand what is added to our food to make it last so long and look so good on grocery store shelves? Can they identify a marketing health claim that's "too good to be true"? Do they know what they need to eat in terms of basic nutrients and why those are so important?

Here are some topics for family discussions to help you get started. As with everything, keep it light and fun for maximum engagement!

- **What are real foods?** I tell kids that real foods grow or live in nature, not a factory. If it's on your plate, and you can imagine where it came from in nature, it's probably a real food. Some real foods can be made with other whole food ingredients, such as whole grain breads or soups and stews. Get your kids to go through the fridge or pantry and identify as many real foods as they can. Make a meal that evening together out of only real food ingredients. Take a trip to the local farmers' market and discuss how the foods available there differ from those available at the supermarket.

- **What are processed foods?** The easiest way to define these for kids is to say processed foods are made in a factory and have lots of unnatural ingredients (things you can't easily identify in nature). Show your kids the ingredient list on processed food and compare that to the one-ingredient whole foods. Explain how chemicals are used to preserve, colour and flavour processed foods. Talk about embracing a "5 or less pronounceable ingredients rule" for processed foods, or the idea of not eating anything if you don't know what it is.

- **What's for dinner?** I encourage parents to combine their praise with a little education. When your children try a new food, praise them for their efforts and let them know why that food matters, by giving them some age-appropriate information. A quick internet search will give you some basic facts you can often leverage to your advantage. For example, when my two were preschoolers, they didn't care much for fish. One night, when serving salmon, I asked them if they knew that the healthy fat in it would make their brains grow. I got out the measuring tape and measured their heads and promised to remeasure after they'd finished. Of course, they were delighted with the post-dinner proof that they'd gotten smarter, and never forgot that healthy fat helps brain development. The added bonus was that they've been eating salmon without flinching ever since.

- **Where did dinner come from?** My time in classrooms has made it clear to me that we are raising a generation of kids who don't realize that the "chicken" in their chicken nuggets is meat from a bird, or that potatoes grow underground. Talk to yours about the importance of knowing where and how their veggies grow and how the animals we eat are raised and fed. Local farmers at community markets love to talk about the care they put into raising their plants and animals — just ask them!

- **Traditional versus conventionally farmed produce:** Kids should know that while it can be cheaper and easier to produce fruits and veggies by using chemicals and GMO seeds, those methods may be harmful to our health and have long-term implications for the planet. We need to teach them to choose carefully and buy local when possible. Take your kids to a local farm or start growing some tomatoes or zucchini in the backyard. Help them to appreciate the work and love that goes into producing natural food, and show them how tasty fresh food can be!

Don't be afraid of these topics. Kids are smart and they want to learn. And most of all, kids want to feel great and be healthy. Who knows, you might just learn a little something new in the process too!

## PICKY EATERS

Most kids are not born with unadventurous palates. Of course, they all go through phases where they are more or less selective in their eating, but as parents, we also inadvertently do a lot to raise our own picky eaters. We feed them the same Fruit Roll-Ups, Goldfish, Cheerios, Bear Paws, granola bars and white pasta for so long that their palates grow accustomed to high-carb, super-sweet, sodium-laden tastes. I made mistakes in this area with my kids, and it took a lot of hard work to reverse them, but it is possible, and it's important. We all want to raise confident eaters who can eat at their friends' homes and new restaurants without stress, and travel to new places and make food part of that experience, don't we? I've worked with some older children who've developed a very restrictive, unhealthy diet and are now paying the price for it socially. The longer habits have been in place, the harder it is to change them, so if you've got a more selective eater, start now — don't wait. That said, if your child is older and set in her picky ways, there's still hope!

Here are my basic principles for raising healthy eaters. If you remember these and use them consistently, you'll see steady improvements.

- **You, as the parent(s), are in charge.** You buy and prepare the food, you choose the restaurants, you set the boundaries — not your kids. Remember this as we go through the other rules and tips, because this really is the underlying foundational rule. They can absolutely make choices, but you set the healthy framework within which that happens.

- **You also set the patterns.** This flows from the first principle. You decide how many cafeteria meals they get a year, how many times a month you will go out to eat and how often they have dessert. If they've never been fed white rice at home, they'll never expect it at home. If they've never been through the McDonald's drive-through with you, they'll never ask you to stop on the way home from hockey.

- **You are not, ever, a short-order cook.** Meet my daily mantra: "This is not a restaurant." Well, come on! It's not, nor should it be. I'm busy and you're busy and it's hard enough work to put one healthy, balanced meal on the table, let alone two or three — if they don't love it, too bad! I know how tempting (and easy) it can be sometimes to just whip up a PB & J in the face of a tantrum at the table, but that's just going to make things worse for all of you. Here's how to handle it without worrying you'll starve them: always provide a healthy side dish or two you know they'll eat, something healthy like sliced apples with almond butter or raw veggies with dip, and a glass of milk or nut milk. They're guaranteed some complex carbs and protein, and you know they aren't going to suffer long-term damage if they don't eat the rest of their dinner. You can stick to your guns and build a consistent approach they will come to rely on. And I promise, they'll make it to the next snack or meal, possibly peckish, but always unscathed!

- **Remain calm and positive at all times.** Easier said then done, right? Here's the thing — I've been steadily working on getting my kids to be more daring eaters for many years now, and I've noticed a pattern. When I pump up a new recipe too much, it's like I'm asking for a negative response. It makes them nervous and highly suspicious. When I just plunk it down, sit down with them and dig in, I'm much less likely to get that initial push-back. When they ask me what's in it, sometimes I tell them, especially if they've had that ingredient before and admitted to liking it, and sometimes I just say, "Yummy goodness and love," and leave it at that until they've had a bite. Reacting to a look of dislike or a gag just escalates things. Instead, I calmly say, "I think it's delicious, and so does your brother, so take one bite, and if you don't want to finish it that's fine, but that's it until the next meal. You can finish your carrots and milk and then be excused." End of discussion. Zero drama.

- **Make meals a family affair.** This is so important for all the social reasons you already know, but also because you have a captive audience at the table. Family dinners provide the perfect opportunity to model healthy habits and talk positively about food. It's a great time to do a little basic nutrition education as well. Don't know why broccoli is great for kids? Google it! They only need to hear once that broccoli has the same bone-building stuff (calcium) in it as milk to remember that fact for life. They have minds like a steel trap, those small people!

- **Don't over-portion.** Kids can get overwhelmed when presented with too full a plate. For younger children, I recommend you stick to 1 tablespoon per year of age for each new food on the plate (i.e., if your child is four, put a maximum of 4 tablespoons of mashed potatoes on the plate).

- **Be shameless, and ask for positive feedback!** Here's an example: "The best feeling for me is when you eat something I've cooked and there's no complaining" or "Boy, do I love it when you tell me you like what I've worked hard to make." You'll be surprised at the snowball effect this can have — your kids love you more than anyone and want to make you feel good. My kids have slowly progressed from eating in silence with no complaints to "This is okay" to "This is good" to "I love this" and, finally, to the proverbial icing on the cake — a standing ovation! They really don't want to disappoint me, so

I rarely get crankiness at mealtimes. The worst I might hear is "It's not my favourite," and I can totally live with that.

• **Praise them for being adventurous and making healthy choices.** It's just like any other taught behaviour — positive reinforcement is huge!

• **Combine your praise with education.** Remember my earlier examples: "Great job eating your salmon. Now your brain has the good fat it needs to grow smarter!" or "Nice job eating the broccoli. It's a superfood. Did you know it can give you superpowers? It will give you the energy you need to run super fast!" The older your kids get, the more information you can give them.

• **Be a great role model.** Treat and feed your body well. If you're having trouble with this, your kids will pick up on it. They see what you eat, but they also see what you don't eat. This can be a good thing or a very bad thing, depending on your choices!

• **Make sure they are hungry when they get to the table.** Cut off healthy snacks at least an hour before meals.

• **Serve new food with a healthy favourite.** This makes new food less overwhelming for kids, and the familiar food ensures they're getting what they need, even if they're only taking a bite or two of the new food.

• **Require regular tasting.** For younger kids, it might be one or two bites, for older ones, it can be more. Tell them it's your job as a parent to help them like as many healthy foods as possible, and because it sometimes takes fifteen to twenty tries for kids to like foods, they need to keep putting them in their mouths and tasting them or they'll never get there. Take the pressure off by telling them you they're not required to like or finish the food yet. They just need to chew and swallow their bite(s) and not make a fuss.

- **Try and try again.** It really does take ten or fifteen tries sometimes before they'll eat and admit to liking a new food. Perseverance is key.

- **It's a continuum — celebrate little victories!** My daughter refused to eat berries for no good reason for about two years. She picked them out of muffins and drove me batty. First, I started serving them in smoothies, then as a side dish at breakfast, and now, she eats them with no complaint in oatmeal and muffins and pretty much everything. One step at a time, at least ten tries on each step! No matter where your kids are on the healthy-eating continuum, there is always a healthier option. Don't get drastic — you will pay the price. If they eat fast food fries, first move to oven-baked fries, then move to sweet potato fries. Don't try to go from zero to sixty — it rarely works! Their taste buds need to adjust to the taste of real food.

- **Make it easier for them to have a victory.** You can do this by downplaying the spices, without removing the flavour. For example, serve a curry with half the spice, and a drizzle of honey to sweeten it slightly, to start. Serve healthy dips and sauces on the side of main dishes. You can even try using small bowls to keep foods from touching if that's a problem for your kids!

- **Use flavours they like to introduce new foods.** For example, if they like maple syrup, toss sweet potatoes in syrup and cinnamon, or flavour their breakfast oats this way.

- **Sneak in the good stuff when you can!** There are lots of easy ways to insert veggies in disguise. My caveat is this: slip them in, but make sure you continue serving whole veggies and fruits with your meals

— you don't want to be sneaking puréed veggies into their food when they're teenagers! And celebrate the secret ingredient! Not telling your kids what's in the food they like is a bad idea — the "if my kids knew what was in here they would never eat it" mentality. Instead, as soon as they admit they like something with hidden veggies in it, get them to guess what the secret ingredient is, so that the next time you serve that veggie you can remind them that they loved it the last time in that recipe you made.

- **Name a healthy dish after them**. Be creative! If they also help you make it, how can they possibly admit to not liking it?

- **Remember to look at the big picture**. It's not what your child eats at a particular meal that matters, it's how he or she does over the course of a day or even over a couple of days. Don't get too caught up in one meal — remain steadfast and offer healthy snacks. If your child is offered only healthy, varied food at snack time and meals, chances are they're getting what they need.

- At the end of the day, here's what I hope you take away from all this talk about healthy family food: it matters, and it's great that you know and prioritize that, and whatever your personal struggles are with feeding your family, you are *not* alone. Dig in and persevere — if you want to raise a happy, healthy kid, then this is just another one of your jobs as a great parent. Give it the same dedication you would other aspects of parenting. Don't expect miracles, but believe that with consistency and dedication you will see steady, positive change.

## SCHOOL LUNCH SOLUTIONS

For many families, school lunches are an area of frustration — packed lunches aren't getting eaten, the cafeteria offerings are less than healthy and parents find themselves in a rut, packing the same meat and cheese sandwich day after day. If you're one of those families, I've got lots of great ideas that will get you packing healthier, more inspired lunches that your kids will actually eat.

Getting out of the sandwich rut isn't nearly as hard as you think. Download my Build-a-Lunch Guide for free (**www.formaclorimer-books.ca/realfood/lunchguide.pdf**) and tape it on the inside of a kitchen cupboard door where everyone can access it easily. This handy chart provides a list of healthy protein, carb and good fat options that you can mix and match. Having a list makes it a lot easier to come up with creative ideas on a rushed morning! Use the Build-a-Lunch Guide along with the healthy lunch ideas below in your weekly meal planning process, then add the ingredients you need to your grocery list so you're always well stocked. If your kids are old enough to pack their own lunches, they can use the guide a resource too. Build away!

### Healthy, Interesting School Lunches Every Day

School lunches don't have to be boring. With just a little planning, they can actually be interesting and pretty much hassle-free. Here are some tips to keep you out of the sandwich rut this year:

- **Think bento box, not lunch box!** Lunch can be so many things besides a sandwich, and a deli box of assorted finger foods is often the easiest way to keeps things fresh and varied. Try whole grain pita, hummus, grapes, carrots and celery; or cubed chicken, white cheddar, sliced apple, whole grain crackers and a mixture of raisins, sunflower and pumpkin seeds, for example. You can buy inexpensive containers with dividers in a variety of sizes for easy deli-box packing.

- **Ice, ice, baby!** Sending frozen food keeps everything in the lunch box cool, and many foods (like frozen healthy muffins or granola bars) will be nicely defrosted by lunchtime. Frozen berries with a little maple syrup and some sunflower seeds in plain yoghurt keep the yoghurt cool all day. A smoothie made with frozen berries and banana will also remain chilly until the lunch bell rings.

- **Heat things up!** A good Thermos will keep things warm for up to five hours and allow you to send almost anything for lunch, including last night's leftovers. Send soup, pasta and sauce, or hot oatmeal with berries and maple syrup — they'll all be nice and warm at lunchtime. Be sure to invest in a good quality Thermos, as the cheaper versions often don't live up to their promises.

- **Become a weekend warrior!** Every Sunday, get your kids involved in prepping some of the basics for the week's lunches. Peel and cut some carrots, celery and cucumber sticks in bulk, for example, and pack in single-serve containers. Make homemade, nut-free granola bars or healthy mini-muffins and freeze two-thirds of the batch for weeks to come. (Try the Chocolate Chip Granola Bars or Good Morning Muffins in my first cookbook, *Real Food for Real Families*. Both are nut-free and freeze well.) Make a batch of chicken noodle or veggie soup and freeze in 1 cup portions. Defrost in the fridge overnight, reheat and send in a Thermos for a delicious hot lunch once or twice a week. I like to use small Mason jars or other lidded glass jars — just be sure to leave a little room at the top for freezer expansion!

- **Don't go nuts!** With nut allergy policies, peanut butter is out, but there are lots of great alternatives for sandwich spreads. Try sunflower seed butter or SunButter (one of my favourites) or another seed butter. Plain cream cheese with apple butter (a natural jam with low sugars) or sliced strawberries makes a great sandwich, and hummus is a yummy, healthy condiment when layered with cucumbers, spinach and tomato.

- **Switch up Your crust!** There are so many ways to make a basic sandwich more interesting. Instead of the usual two slices of bread, why not try another whole grain option: waffles (make and freeze on the weekend), pitas, tortillas, rice cakes, and pancakes or crepes can all make fun envelopes for the fillings.

- **Pack a protein punch!** Don't send a carb-filled lunch box. Remember, refined carbs like white flours and sugars will just provide your kids with a quick blood-sugar high followed by a corresponding low, making it difficult for them to focus and learn. Send good carbs like whole grains, veggies and fruits, but pair them with some protein and a little healthy fat for a longer-lasting, steadier release of energy. Check the Build-a-Lunch Guide for easy lunch-box proteins and fats to pack alongside healthy carbs.

- **Send some lunch-box love!** A little love note, a kids' joke or trivia fact or a reminder about a fun after-school activity can make an anxious child's day, especially in the early days of September. Make a few up on little cards on the weekend, keep them in a drawer in the kitchen and toss them into the lunch box once in a while to remind your wee ones you're thinking of them even when you're not together!

- **Start their day right and pack light!** It's very common for small children just starting school to be overwhelmed at lunchtime and not eat much lunch at all. Expect that, and talk to them about it if their lunch comes home uneaten. Sometimes they can't figure out how to open the containers, other times they can't eat fast enough (they'll only have about fifteen to twenty minutes at most public schools) or maybe they get distracted socially and forget to eat. Packing a lighter lunch sets them up for success. If you pack less, they're less likely to be overwhelmed, more likely to eat and you'll have the opportunity to praise them when they get home. Slowly add more food as they get better at finishing most of what you send. Be realistic, though; for many parents it's a continuing struggle. There are still some days when my eleven-year-old daughter, for whatever reason, just doesn't eat enough at school. Because I know that's a possibility, I make sure she's as well prepared as possible by feeding her a terrific breakfast every morning, and I require her to eat any uneaten items from her lunch after school.

- **Set cafeteria rules!** If your goal is to send a packed lunch most days, I recommend setting some boundaries at the beginning of the school year about the number of times your child will visit the cafeteria to prevent begging down the road. You might agree on once a month, or twice a year, or never, but if you don't decide upfront, those cafeteria menus that come home in their backpacks will become a thorn in your backside! Set a healthy pattern early, and by the time they're in grade 2, they'll stop asking altogether.

## School Lunch Ideas

- Mini-pizza on a whole wheat English muffin with real cheese

- Whole grain tortilla with cream cheese and sliced strawberries or pears, roll-up style

- Sliced, roasted chicken or nitrate-free sandwich meat with toppings in a whole grain pita, on bread or on a bagel

- Turkey pinwheels: whole grain tortilla, nitrate-free turkey, hummus and spinach rolled up and cut into pinwheels

- Egg salad on whole grain: 2 hard-boiled eggs mixed with 1 tsp plain yoghurt, 1/2 tsp mustard, salt and black pepper

- Sunflower seed butter, honey and banana sandwich on whole grain

- Whole grain pasta salad with whatever veggies your child likes, chopped cheese, meat or hard-boiled egg and healthy salad dressing

- Quesadilla or burrito-style wrap on whole grain tortilla with black beans, avocado, salsa, Greek yoghurt, hummus, shredded cheese, veggies (whatever they like)

- Deli plate of assorted "finger foods": cubed chicken, cheese, hummus or tzatziki dip, baby carrots, cherry tomatoes, olives and whole grain crackers

- Cream cheese and apple butter on a whole grain bagel

- Sunflower seed butter and apple butter sandwich

- Whole grain pasta with tomato sauce and feta or cubed chicken in a Thermos

- Low-sodium veggie or other soup with whole grain crackers (add chicken or beans for protein)

- Veggie chili in a Thermos with whole grain crackers or roll

- Whole grain waffles cut in strips with yoghurt for dipping

- Veggie and hummus wraps (tortillas or whole wheat pitas)

- Whole wheat pita triangles with bean dip and raw veggies

- Fruit salad with yoghurt and nut-free granola

- Fruit kebabs or meat, cheese and veggie kebabs

- Other ideas? Add them to your list!

# CHAPTER 21

## Keeping It Real

## MINDFUL EATING AND CRAVINGS

Food should always be pleasurable — it might surprise you, but I really believe that. In fact, I think we should practise "joyful eating" (as corny as it might sound) whenever possible. Once you really value your wellness, healthy eating becomes joyous. Putting good quality, nourishing, tasty food in your mouth feels great.

That said, sometimes eating not-so-perfect food can also be joyous. If you choose to eat something not-so-real you know you won't second-guess later on, it's joyful eating. An anniversary, holiday or birthday dinner celebrated with family and friends might involve richer foods, sweets and drinks — if it's a true celebration, it's probably joyful eating even if it's not technically healthy, because you won't regret it the next day. Just keep in mind that, while you might not regret the first slice of birthday cake, you'll probably wish you hadn't helped yourself to a second. And while a big slice of cake and a glass or two of wine on your birthday might be joyful eating, it's not nearly as joyous when it's wolfed down with the *Real Housewives of Orange County*.

The trick is to be mindful. You need to think before you eat, as simple as that sounds. If you don't, you'll find it's surprisingly easy to mindlessly consume a load of unhealthy, empty calories. Get into the habit of asking yourself a few questions (although it's probably best not to do this out loud) before you eat anything: "Am I actually hungry?" and "Could I make a better choice?" and maybe "How will I feel after eating this food?" Ninety per cent of the time, just thinking before you eat will lead to a good decision. If it doesn't, at least you consciously chose it. Remember, the first bite tastes the same as the last but involves a lot less guilt, so enjoy a few bites and get on with the business of being you.

As long as we're keeping it real though, the truth is that sometimes even a healthy snack won't satisfy the craving. When this is the case, you're eating for another reason altogether — it could be boredom or loneliness (my personal Achilles heel), depression, stress, anxiety or any number of emotions. Think of your food as fuel, not entertainment or a distraction. If you need entertaining, call a friend, go for a walk, rent a movie or buy a new book — don't eat.

Sometimes, no matter what you do, you just can't shake a craving. This is when you need a reliable, fail-safe distraction. The most effective solution is to remove yourself from the temptation — go outside for a walk or to a friend's, hop in the bath or simply go to bed. Whatever it is, practise it over and over until it becomes your habitual response to unexplained, unsinkable cravings. If after all that you still just need to have it, then have it and then let it be! You're human, after all. Follow it up with a healthy next meal and move on.

## Staying Motivated

When you feel your motivation dipping, or you've hit a plateau, reread the first few chapters of this book, and look over this list to help you stay on track:

- Take it one healthy meal at a time. It can be overwhelming, especially in the beginning, to consider that you will be eating this way for the rest of your life. Remember, once you reach your goal there will be more room for moderation and the 80/20 rule will allow lots of flexibility.

- Commit to just three days of clean eating. It's not too overwhelming, and in my experience, this will get you right back on track as you're reminded of how easy it is and how awesome you feel.

- What will make this time different from the last weight-loss effort is not that you'll stop slipping up, because that's just part of being human. What will be different is how you react to less-than-perfect days. It's the "being able to get back on track" bit that makes you a healthy eater. That's the part you are now great at.

- Remember that if the "outside mirror" isn't reflecting what you'd like to see yet, the "inside mirror" probably is. In a week where you don't lose on the outside, you've still gained on the inside — your vitamin and mineral bank account is full, your energy is up, your digestive system is running like a fine-tuned machine and your immune system is booming!

- Make a list of the most important reasons for making permanent changes and achieving your healthy weight, and keep it with you as a reminder when you are feeling discouraged. Remind yourself of how far you've already come. Where you would be if you hadn't become a healthy eater? Probably heavier, less energetic and sick more often. How would you feel, mentally and physically, if you went back to your old habits?

- Get moving! Sometimes, a little change in your exercise patterns can be enough to lift you right back up. Pick up a new pair of sweats that make you feel great, choose a new class to try, or download a motivating, upbeat mix of tunes or an e-book to enjoy while you work out.

### Stress Management.

We all talk the talk when it comes to stress. It's almost a badge of honour in many circles to be "so busy you haven't slept in days." And while we might dabble in yoga, exercise or even meditation, those stress management activities are the first thing to go when the going gets tough. I know — I've been there. I talked the talk for years.

But now (thankfully), it's my job to teach you to walk the walk. In my experience, when people *really* understand what's actually happening to their bodies under stress and the serious damage it can cause, they're a lot less proud of their crazy life, and a lot more motivated to stop sweating the small stuff and, sometimes, make some bigger changes. Here's the dangerous truth about stress, and some of my most practical strategies for regaining a little of that elusive balance.

Stress, whether it's physical (like illness or sleep deprivation), emotional (like grief or anger) or mental (think deadlines and complex assignments), is an essential and unavoidable aspect of human life. While we tend to think of it as a negative, it's often a very positive force, motivating us to complete tasks and work efficiently. However, when we have too much stress in our lives and don't manage it properly, its short-term physiological effects can turn into chronic problems for our bodies, and it becomes dangerous.

Physical, mental and emotional stress all cause the same physiological response, called "fight or flight," which releases a flood of stress hormones, including adrenalin and cortisol, into your bloodstream. These trigger your body to prepare for emergency action and deal with that threat — by fighting it off or getting away to safety.

Here's an extreme example of the fight or flight response in action. Imagine a caveman who goes out hunting. He's relaxed when he heads out, but becomes anxious when he sees a sabre-toothed tiger. He automatically goes into the fight or flight response: his heart rate increases, muscles tighten, blood pressure rises, breath quickens and senses sharpen. At the same time, the systems his body perceives as "non-essential" to dealing with the threat, such as his digestion, are suppressed. These physical changes increase his strength and stamina, speed his reaction time and enhance his focus — preparing him to either fight or flee from the danger at hand.

Now, as I see it, there are three possible outcomes to this encounter. The caveman kills the tiger and relaxes as the danger has passed; he decides the risk is too high and flees to safety instead of fighting the tiger, relaxing when he's home free; or the caveman gets eaten, in which case he's also relaxed in pretty short order. The point is, the stress response is designed to be short-term and to be followed pretty quickly by the "calm after the storm," during which cortisol drops and both the heightened and compromised body systems return to normal.

The problem is, the relaxation stage is just not happening enough in our busy, modern lives. Most people I work with say their life is either a constant series of stressful events or that they just feel like they're under an umbrella of stress 24-7. In either case, their cortisol is going up and staying up more often and for longer than it's meant to.

Cortisol is an important hormone with many essential functions, including regulating glucose metabolism, blood pressure, insulin and the immune response. In healthy amounts, and in the short-term, it's helpful. But if it's chronically elevated, cortisol causes increased belly fat. This is associated with a lot of health problems, including something called "metabolic syndrome," characterized by a triad of symptoms: high blood pressure, high blood sugar and high triglycerides.

Chronic stress disrupts nearly every system in your body. Along with increasing your risk of developing type 2 diabetes, heart disease and stroke, it can affect your immune and thyroid function, your sleep patterns, your brain, your fertility and speed up aging. It encourages your body to store carbohydrate as fat, instead of burning it for energy, making it easier to gain weight and harder to lose weight if you're stressed. Sound like something you should work harder at managing?

Imagine you have a cup designed to hold cortisol, but it can hold only so much, and when that cup starts to overflow you start to get sick. Everyone's cup is a slightly different size, and the problem is, you won't know how big your cup is until it overflows. One of your jobs over the course of your lifetime, if you want to stay well, is to try to reduce the amount of cortisol going into your cup. Life hands us lots of stress and related cortisol that we've got little choice but to accept — we get sick, loved ones die, relationships end and jobs get overwhelming. But there are lots of experiences that we have active control over, at least in terms of how we react. If we consistently choose to react in a negative way, worrying about things outside of our control, holding grudges, getting angry about things that aren't worth getting angry about and reacting to people who aren't worth reacting to, we're dumping a whole lot of unnecessary cortisol into that cup.

Once we realize that those challenging experiences and people in our lives have the potential to negatively affect our health, we might just start reacting differently. Everyone has "cortisol-jackers" in their life, whether they're social or professional acquaintances, strangers or family. Are you willing to let someone else's behaviour and choices affect your health? When you find yourself in the presence of a cortisol-jacker, it's often helpful to recite one of my favourite Polish proverbs (all right, it's my only Polish proverb) — "Not my circus, not my monkeys." Don't get caught up in other people's drama, don't get irate when there's a traffic accident or the person in front of you at the store forgot to put something in her cart. Take a breath and repeat, "Not my circus, not my monkeys."

Here's some great news — even when stress is severe and long-term and the kind we can't just shake off, we can still do something proactive to reduce the negative impacts of cortisol. It's easy and cheap and you can do it just about anywhere — it's called deep breathing. Here's how it works: when a situation presents itself and you feel yourself getting stressed, stop doing what you are doing and force yourself to take ten long, slow, deep breaths (not the kind where your chest puffs out, the kind where your belly swells). You'll instantly feel calmer, but more important, you've tricked your body into thinking the threat has passed by changing your breathing patterns and reversing that domino effect of stress-driven symptoms. When your breathing slows, your heartbeat slows, your blood pressure decreases, your muscles relax and your cortisol goes down!

By now, you're probably convinced. Stress management actually matters. It helps you manage your cortisol and mood and just generally cope better through periods of long-term stress. The healthiest people out there are also just a little bit selfish — they realize that it's not a bad thing to put themselves first, and they make a point of doing what's necessary to keep their balance. They make and take time to shop, cook and pack food, exercise and sleep. They also prioritize fun, whether it's with family or friends. Sometimes that takes time away from their kids or spouse or job, but they're okay with that, because what kind of parent, spouse or employee are they going to be if they're stressed out, sick and resentful?

So, do yourself a favour: consider saying no once in a while, and don't just pencil in exercise, kitchen time or coffee with friends, use a Sharpie! Schedule the other stuff around it, and make it happen. Just like everything else, the more you do it, the easier it gets. And stop sweating the small stuff!

### Sleep

Poor sleep also affects cortisol. If you're a parent, your number-one sleep disruptor is probably your wakeful wee ones, but plenty of other things, like anxiety, job stress and shiftwork can all make it hard to get to sleep and stay asleep. It's well worth putting in some work to get both the hours and quality of sleep that you need. Not only does a bad sleep pattern create additional cortisol and increase carb cravings, it also wreaks havoc with your "hunger hormones," making it even harder to stick to healthy choices during the day. When you are sleep deprived, your body makes more ghrelin (the hormone that signals it's time to eat) and less leptin (the one that tells you you've had enough), and that's a surefire recipe for weight gain.

Go to bed fifteen or thirty minutes earlier, incorporate regular exercise earlier in your day, install blackout shades, wear earplugs, take the TV out of your room or start a nighttime ritual of herbal tea, a hot bath or reading before bed. If those suggestions don't work, get help from a professional. It's worth it.

## Exercise

I can't emphasize enough the importance of enjoyable, moderate exercise for lifelong wellness and weight maintenance. Notice how I said "enjoyable" and "moderate"? Torturous extreme activity lasts about as long as restrictive and extreme dieting. Embrace moderation and find something you love that you will continue to do often. You don't need to set aside large chunks of time for exercise to reap the benefits. If you can't fit in a scheduled workout, get more active throughout the day in simple ways — take the stairs instead of the elevator, play outside with the kids, rev up your household chores or walk the dog a little farther and a little faster.

No matter what your current weight, getting and staying active can help prevent or manage a wide range of health problems and concerns, including stroke, metabolic syndrome, type 2 diabetes and depression. Exercise also improves mood and sleep and can give you a chance to unwind, enjoy the outdoors or simply engage in an activity with others that make you happy. So, take a dance class, hit the hiking trails, pick up your dusty racket or join a soccer team. Find a physical activity you enjoy, and just do it. If you get bored, try something new.

Aim to move your body every day, increasing your endurance gradually. Remember to check with your doctor before starting a new exercise program, especially if you have any health concerns.

## Vacations

There is really nothing worse than coming home from a vacation to pants that no longer fit or nursing a vacation "hangover" caused by an excess of unhealthy food and booze. With just a little effort, you really can have a fantastic trip and maintain balance. It's not about being perfect, it's about being mindful. Planning is essential for vacation success, especially when you are planning for a bit of less-than-perfect eating!

Be prepared, choose your treats wisely and move your body, and you'll find you come back relatively unscathed. Here are a few of my favourite tips:

- **Pack your snacks!** A container of natural almond or peanut butter, a bag of raw almonds, brown rice cakes, pre-portioned homemade granola bars and fruit can keep you on track between meals. If you can't get to a grocery store at your destination, bring snacks with you. A box of your favourite herbal tea can provide a relaxing alternative to a sugary drink or alcoholic beverage.

- **Exercise every day.** Walking counts! Buy a pedometer or download an app to track your steps and aim for a minimum of 10,000 a day. If you're strolling the beach, hitting local attractions or even shopping, you'll be amazed at how fast you'll get there. If there are classes or organized sports offered where you are going, take part in these too.

- **Skip the white stuff.** The easiest way to keep your calorie intake in check is to commit to no refined flours or sugars while you are away. That means no bread, crackers, cakes or cookies. If you have grains, be sure to keep them whole, such as oatmeal or brown rice.

- **Salad days!** When I'm away, I get into a routine of veggies, fruit and lean protein, no grains, for breakfast and lunch. For example, breakfast might be poached eggs with steamed or sautéed greens, broiled tomato and a side of fruit, and lunch might be salad with loads of veggies topped with grilled chicken or fish. Always choose a vinaigrette over a creamy dressing (many salad bars will allow you to mix your own with oil and vinegar). Lighter breakfast and lunch balances out a splurge at dinner.

- **Make your dessert fruit, unless it's really worth it.** One ice cream or slice of key lime pie isn't going to break you, but a daily dessert will. Choose to have it when it's really worth it, but choose fruit or just share a bite when it's not.

- **Drink wisely, my friends!** All alcoholic beverages are not created equal. Choose lower-calorie drinks such as wine, light beer or vodka sodas over mixed fruity concoctions. Cut your wine calories in half by mixing soda water and a slice of lemon with white wine. Drink one glass of water between every alcoholic beverage. You'll consume less and feel better.

- **Beware of buffets.** Circle the buffet once or twice before choosing your food. Take a small plate, fill at least half of it with salad or veggies and don't go back for seconds.

- **Grab and go.** I regularly pocket fruit and hard-boiled eggs at the breakfast buffet for a healthy mid-morning snack. The snack bars at all-inclusives are usually *deadly* and should be avoided at all costs!

- **Make special requests.** For example, ask the waiter *not* to bring a bread basket, ask the omelette station if they can prepare an oil-free, mostly egg-white omelette with extra veggies, ask the bartender to make your white wine a spritzer or ask if you can have the grilled fish without the sauce and your salad dressing on the side. If you don't ask, they won't offer, but in my experience they will almost always accommodate you.

- **Have fun!** Don't beat yourself up if you're not perfect. Do your best. There's nothing that a week or two of clean eating can't undo upon your return.

### Travelling for Work

Going on the road or out of town for work might make healthy eating more challenging, but with a little planning it's always doable. Take control over whatever meals and snacks you can, and just do your best with the rest:

- **Pack your breakfasts.** Pre-measure and package quick/instant oats, cinnamon, ground flax, nuts and a little stevia or a little brown sugar in zip-top bags or heatproof containers. In your hotel room, add hot water (run a pot through the coffeemaker, without the coffee), let it sit, toss in some fruit, and enjoy.

- **Pack your snacks.** If you're travelling within the country, you can pack most of the healthy snacks you eat at home, including almond butter, raw almonds, brown rice cakes, homemade muffins or granola bars and fruit. If you're going across the border you need to be more careful, but can often find a convenience store or grocery store near your hotel to stock up on these foods.

- **If you're driving all day, pack a cooler.** Hard-boiled eggs, fruit, precut raw veggies and hummus and premade salads made from longer-lasting ingredients like quinoa, cabbage (coleslaw), brown rice or rice noodles travel well.

- **Before you leave (or better yet, before you book), check out your hotel online.** Is there a gym or a pool? If so, pack your gear. Is there a kitchenette or at least a fridge and microwave in your room so you can prepare some of your own food? Can you scope out the restaurant menu in advance and identify some better choices? If nothing looks very healthy, call or email the hotel and ask how difficult it will be to order off the menu (i.e., a salad with a grilled chicken breast or fillet of fish, or fruit with oatmeal or poached eggs for breakfast). Most hotels recognize the importance of being flexible, but if they're not willing to bend the menu, ask for the names of restaurants close to the hotel, check those menus out and find out where the closest grocery store is.

- **Manage client dinners as best you can.** Remember the "joyful eating" thing? Just because you're at a restaurant doesn't mean it's a time of celebration, and if you're regularly at work functions, chances are you'd rather be somewhere else and there is nothing joyous about it. If you have the option, choose the restaurant instead of letting someone else do that, so you can opt for something with healthier choices. Order a salad with dressing on the side (vinaigrettes tend to be a better bet) and some grilled (not fried) protein on top, or grilled protein with rice and vegetables. Or choose a small veggie pizza or pasta and ask for half the cheese or noodles and twice the veggies. Skip the bread basket and drink water if you can. Have some fruit for dessert or politely decline. Do your best, and you'll feel that much better when you get back to the hotel.

## Holidays and Special Occasions

When you have a big celebration or holiday coming up, you need a strategy that will allow you to enjoy the event fully without the corresponding guilt. Maybe you plan to enjoy dessert but stick to water, or look forward to turkey and wine but skip the bread basket and get in a little extra exercise that day. Here are a few of my best tips to help you get through the holiday season unscathed:

- **Remember, it's a holi"day" not a holi"month"!** There is absolutely no reason to indulge at every event you attend in December, for example. That — not one or two celebratory dinners — is what adds up to all the extra pounds come January. It's an excuse to overindulge and gain weight only if you decide it is.

- **Practise mindful eating.** Think about what is going in your mouth. If it doesn't look unbelievably divine and unique, why eat it? Most of the foods served during the holidays are not really that special. Those chips and dip, chocolates and cheese plates will all be available tomorrow, and even next month. You are not being deprived of something if you can choose to have it at another time! Ask yourself, "Is this worth it?"

- **Bring something healthy to the table.** The hostess will appreciate it and you'll have something good to eat. Think salads, fruit trays, hummus and veggies.

- **Don't go out hungry.** If you haven't eaten in the last few hours, eat a good snack combining complex carbs, protein and healthy fat. It will keep your blood sugar and willpower intact.

- **For uniquely seasonal foods, indulge mindfully!** For example, your mom's pumpkin pie. She makes it but once a year and it's delicious. The first piece you eat will be as delicious and decadent as you remember, and you'll eat it with joy as it reminds you of happy holidays past. I'm willing to bet, though, that the second helping won't come with those warm feelings attached — just a whole bunch of guilt and indigestion.

- **Grazing at the buffet isn't joyful eating.** The best buffet strategy is to take a good look first, figure out what is healthy and really worth it and then put that on your plate and enjoy it thoroughly. And don't go back for seconds!

- **All alcohol is not created equal.** A glass of eggnog has about 380 calories, while a glass of white wine has only 100. A fancy cocktail or hot toddy can have upward of 500 calories. If you love a special seasonal drink, savour one then move on to the more calorie-friendly ones (the most friendly of all being water) for the remainder of the season. Someone will be serving eggnog next year. It's often not the calories in alcohol that lead to weight gain, but rather the loss of inhibitions and willpower that go along with it. We lose our ability to make good choices and eventually end up with a plateful of junk to wash down. Practise safe drinking! Volunteer to be the designated driver. Or drink alcohol only with a meal. Limit yourself to one or two drinks and then switch to sparkling water.

- **Exercise daily**. You will inevitably eat a little more than average many days of the holidays. The best way to counter this is to move your body, so if you exercise most days you'll be ahead of the game when the decorations come down.

## Moderation and Maintenance

By now I hope you truly understand that focusing on wellness rather than appearance is a more effective approach in terms of long-term weight-loss success. You are feeling and looking terrific right now as a result of the new eating habits you have developed through this program. If you start falling back into old patterns, not only will you regain the weight, but you'll reverse all the progress you've made in preventing long-term health problems and will start to feel the way you did before you started making changes.

Losing even small amounts of body weight can lead to big health rewards in terms of lower blood pressure, cholesterol, blood-sugar levels, inflammation, energy levels and your ability to manage stress. Weight and wellness maintenance requires regular exercise, eating healthy food most of the time, some self-monitoring and a commitment to carving out the time you need to make it happen.

The following habits are essential to weight maintenance success:

- **Continue your exercise program.** Studies suggest that it takes thirty to sixty minutes of moderately intense physical activity daily to maintain weight loss (i.e., fast walking or swimming).

- **Practise healthy meal and snack planning.** Even when you are not following a strict meal plan, this is the key to eating well for life. You can't make healthy choices if the food is not in your kitchen.

- **Combine complex carbs, healthy protein and fat.** Focus on whole, nutrient-dense foods and keep eating seven to ten servings of fruits and veggies a day. Stick to the 80/20 (or better!) rule when it comes to the not-so-perfect foods, and even then, make the best choices you can. Maintain variety in your whole foods, and remember that no one food offers all the nutrients you need.

- **Know and avoid personal food traps that cause you to overeat.** Know which situations can trigger out-of-control eating for you. The best way to identify food traps and emotionally triggered eating is to keep a journal. For as long as you find it helpful, write down what you eat, how much you eat, when you eat, how you're feeling and how hungry you are. After a while, you should see some patterns emerge. Once you know these patterns and triggers, you can plan ahead and develop a strategy for how you'll handle these types of situations. This will help you understand and stay in control of your eating behaviours.

- **Monitor your weight regularly.** People who do this are more successful in keeping off the pounds, as this allows them to detect small weight gains before they become larger. If you hate the scale, use a pair of fitted pants as a measuring tool. Go back to your meal plan if those pants are too tight or you're up five pounds or more from your goal weight. Stay on it until you are back where you should be.

- **Be consistent.** Sticking to your healthy-weight plan during the week, on the weekends and amidst vacation and holidays increases your chances of long-term success.

- **Create a support network.** Get your spouse, family members and friends on board when it comes to making healthy choices and being active.

- **Weight maintenance gets easier over time.** After two to five years, the odds of keeping the weight off increase greatly. Staying at a healthy weight does take planning and effort, but the rewards are great.

Now here are the basic rules of achieving and maintaining your own lifelong simple balance — basically a summary of everything in this program. None of these are absolute, and there will be times when you choose, or need, to break them. When you get to a place where you are following these most of the time, you'll be able to say with confidence that you are eating a healthy diet and don't have to constantly worry about your weight or wellness.

- **Eat at least 80 per cent of your food as whole, real, unprocessed foods.** Vegetables and fruits, nuts and seeds, clean lean proteins, whole grains and healthy fats.

- **Eat mostly plants.** People who eat mostly plants weigh less and live longer. Can you argue with that? Aim for seven to ten servings of fruits and veggies a day.

- **Eliminate refined grains and sugars — no "white stuff" in your daily food.** Whole grains are brown, not white, and added sugars contribute to weight gain, blood-sugar imbalances and an increased risk of a whole host of diseases.

- **Eliminate unhealthy, processed fats.** Hydrogenated, partially hydrogenated and trans fats have no place in a clean, healthy body. Read labels and avoid these. The less processed food you eat, the easier this is to accomplish.

- **Enjoy healthy fat in moderation.** Nuts and seeds and many plant oils provide healthy fat, but too many of these will hinder weight loss. Keep it in balance: a teaspoon of healthy oil on a salad, a small handful of nuts as a snack, a tablespoon of nuts/seeds as a salad or oatmeal topper.

- **Eat a minimum of one serving of dark, leafy greens daily.**

Remember, we get some healthy fat from dark, leafy green veggies, and they are low in calories, nutrient-dense and full of fibre.

- **Reduce your dairy and processed or industrially farmed meat.** If your diet is real and varied, you'll get easily absorbable calcium from your plant intake and good quality protein from your veggies, whole grains and naturally raised animal products.

- **Exercise regularly, but have fun doing it.** Find something you enjoy, and set some goals for yourself. Too many of us dislike what we are doing as exercise and find it a chore, or do the same treadmill or elliptical workout daily with no results. Challenge yourself!

- **Sleep, and sleep well.** Proper sleep can add years to your life, keep you on track with weight loss and energize you for the day. Don't underestimate the power of sleep; it's key to your simple balance.

- **Be just a wee bit selfish.** You'll need to make the time to shop and cook your healthy food, sleep, manage your stress and exercise — nobody else can do that but you.

- **Don't sweat the small stuff!** All that small stuff jacks up your cortisol and can negatively impact your weight and health! Is it worth it? Nope. In times of significant stress, ask for help.

# CHAPTER 22

## FAQ

**How much does 1 cup of dry quinoa yield?** 1 cup dry = about 3 cups cooked.

**How much does 1 cup dry green lentils yield?** 1 cup dry = about 2 1/2 cups cooked.

**I'm thinking about buying a Community Shared Agriculture (CSA) farm box this year. Do you have any recommendations, or things I should look for?** Make sure you buy the right size for your family. Know that with most CSAs, you get what you get. You'll get *really* good at cooking root veggies. Personally, I find a smaller half share is plenty for my four-person family. Many CSAs offer shares of foods other than veggies, like pastured eggs, fruits and meats and add-ons of local products like honey and maple syrup. If you're interested in more than veggies, research the variety offered by local CSAs before choosing one.

**I have tried to find whole wheat pastry flour at my local grocery store but can't seem to locate it. I'm wondering if there is a special place to find this?** A bulk food store will usually carry whole wheat pastry flour as will most natural food stores.

**My husband brought home salmon today from the grocery store. It is labelled Atlantic salmon. How do I know if it is farmed or wild?** It's farmed. There is no wild Atlantic salmon fishery right now — there is a moratorium/ban on. Unless you caught it yourself in a river, it's farmed.

**What's the difference between extra-firm, firm and soft tofu? Does it matter what kind you buy, and does it need to be organic?** "Firm," "extra-firm" or "soft" refers to the consistency and texture of the tofu. I recommend firm or extra-firm tofu for stir-fries, breakfast scrambles or whenever you want the tofu to retain its shape (like tofu "steaks" on the grill). Soft tofu is great for puddings, smoothies, or in baked goods. When a recipe calls for regular tofu, it's usually referring to firm or extra-firm. Use soft when that is specified, because substituting in firm usually won't work well. It doesn't have to be organic, but your tofu should at least be made with non-GMO soybeans. Check the label. If it's organic, you know it's non-GMO, otherwise the ingredient list should specify non-GMO soybeans.

**I don't love cilantro, and you use it often in your recipes. Can you recommend a substitute?** Yes, the same amount of fresh parsley usually subs in well for cilantro in my recipes.

**Can I use regular paprika in the place of smoked paprika in your recipes?** Absolutely. You either love or really don't love smoked paprika, in my experience. If you're not a lover, use regular paprika and you'll lose the smoky flavour but keep the zip.

**Can I eat Mary's (gluten-free) crackers or other gluten-free breads and crackers on the Cleanstart week? What about Ezekiel or other sprouted breads?** Nope. Crackers and breads are a slippery slope for most and better just left out of a clean-eating week where you are resetting habits and kickstarting weight loss. After a Cleanstart week, you can incorporate them in moderation.

**Can I use protein powder on your program?** After the Cleanstart week, "clean" protein powders are fine in moderation. That just means a protein powder with no weird or artificial ingredients or a ton of sugar. You can choose from whey, hemp or other vegetarian protein — whatever you prefer.

**How long do homemade salad dressings last in the fridge?** Five to seven days, but you can usually freeze them if you're cooking for one or two and don't think you'll get through a big batch that quickly.

**Do you have any ideas for quick, "clean" marinades for grilling fish and meat?** Try lemon juice, oil, salt, black pepper and garlic (just don't marinate fish in this for more than a few minutes before grilling or it will break down); Bragg soy seasoning with crushed garlic and black bean sauce or sesame oil; fresh herb pesto (blitz cilantro/parsley/basil/chives — basically whatever herbs you've got — with a little olive oil and maybe some balsamic vinegar in the food processor); or lime juice, garlic, cumin and chili for a Mexican-inspired marinade.

**Can I freeze brown rice? What about quinoa and quinoa salads?** Yes! Brown rice and quinoa both freeze well and are great to have on hand in 1/2 cup portions to go with a soup or chili at lunchtime. You can freeze quinoa salads, but know that upon defrosting the texture of the veggies (such as tomatoes) might change a bit. They'll still taste great, though!

**Can I chew gum while following Cleanstart?** I'm not that extreme — if it gets you through the week, go for it!

**Should I keep taking any supplements and medications I was taking**

**before I started the program?** If you've had them prescribed or been advised by a medical or other qualified health practitioner to use medications or certain supplements, continue doing so. As your diet improves it may be the case that those medications and supplements can be reduced or altered, but of course that is something you will need to discuss with your treating practitioner.

**Can I take Advil and other painkillers if I have a headache?** Of course — ibuprofen and other painkillers won't impact weight loss, and headaches stink, so if you need them, go ahead and use them as directed on the product packaging.

**Is it safe or healthy to have boiled eggs daily?** Yes. Unless you've been advised specifically by a treating medical or health practitioner to avoid eggs, go for it. In recent years, eggs have been cleared of the bad rap they once had. Don't avoid the yolks; that's where the vitamins and minerals are. The whites are mostly protein, which is why I sometimes suggest you add 1/4 cup extra egg whites to your brekkie — more protein will fill you up and fuel you for longer.

**Wild rice versus brown rice, short grain versus long grain — does it matter?** As long as your rice is whole grain, it doesn't much matter if it's wild or brown or black, or short or long grain. Even brown basmati is fine. As long as it's whole grain (not white), you're good. You're looking for the fibre and the nutrients you get from whole grain rice. Try a few varieties and find what you like! Personally, I prefer short-grain brown or brown basmati (Lundberg makes great versions of both).

**How long do hard-boiled eggs last in the fridge?** One week. I label mine right on the shell with the date with a Sharpie after they cool.

**Juicing is very popular these days. Are you a fan?** While fresh veggie juice is technically "program-friendly," I prefer whole fruits and

222

veggies to juiced versions because the fibre is retained, so it's a bit easier on your blood sugar and is supportive of healthy digestion. I'm a bigger fan of smoothies than I am of juices, because the fibre/pulp is retained in the blender.

**I'm worried about sugar cravings when I cut out processed stuff and treats — any tips?** Yes, get yourself a really nicely flavoured herbal tea. In my opinion, the best cleanse-friendly tea to curb a sugar craving is the President's Choice brand Chocolatey Chai with a splash of almond milk. Second runner-up for me is Celestial Seasonings Bengal Spice. There are lots of options out there, though, so get a selection and develop an evening tea ritual like Oprah's. Apple butter with a little almond butter on a brown rice cake is also often enough to nip a craving in the bud, if you're not a fan of tea.

**Should I cook the Buddha Burgers before freezing or form them into patties and freeze them raw?** I recommend you cook them first, then freeze them with a square of parchment or waxed paper between the patties. This makes it easy to grab one and heat it up for a delicious, healthy fast food meal on a busy evening!

**I love the Buddha Bowls but it's only me for dinner most nights — can I freeze the leftovers?** Yes! The sauce and the shredded veggies both freeze well. Rice freezes well too, so you can have the whole meal frozen and ready to assemble when the craving strikes!

**We have a nut allergy in the family and need to avoid any products with a "may contain nuts" warning. Can you recommend a tahini (sesame seed paste) that fits the bill?** The NutSmith Tahini made by YUM Foods in Windsor, Nova Scotia, does not have a "may contain nuts" warning. You can get it at grocery stores in Atlantic Canada (natural food section) or natural food stores. If you are outside Atlantic Canada, ask for a recommendation at your local health food store.

**Your recipes often call for fresh herbs like cilantro, basil or parsley. Can I substitute dried?** Yes, you can pretty much always substitute 1 teaspoon of dried for every tablespoon of fresh herbs in a recipe, but know this: it probably won't taste nearly as awesome. **A tip for fresh herbs:** Keep them fresher longer by storing bunches with the roots down in a Mason jar of water in your fridge, and just snip or tear off what you need as you go. If you're going to use only a small bit of your bunch, you can always purée the rest with a little olive oil and then freeze it in tablespoon-sized portions on a plate covered in waxed paper. Pop the frozen spoonfuls off and store them in a freezer-safe, labelled container for use in future recipes.

**Can I have wine? Please?** Outside of the Cleanstart week, if you can have a glass of wine and not get derailed on food choices as a result, go for it. If it's a trigger for reduced willpower and not-so-great food choices, hold off.

**What is your take on canned tuna? Is it okay to use? Also, for sandwiches, with chicken, tuna, et cetera, do you recommend using mayo or something else to moisten the sandwich?** I recommend you eat tuna no more than once per week because of toxicity levels in that fish. When buying tuna, look for canned light tuna or albacore tuna (troll- or pole-caught), which tend to have lower levels of mercury than other types of tuna. In terms of sandwich spreads, Greek yoghurt, homemade tzatziki and avocado are all great options. I also like to use hummus or another type of bean dip as a condiment in veggie and chicken sandwiches. If using mayo, choose an olive oil–based version and make sure there are no junky fats in it. Read labels. If you're not sure about an ingredient, just Google it.

**Where do I get toasted sesame oil?** At your local health food store and probably any Asian food store. That said, you can always use regular sesame oil in its place, which you can get in the Asian food section of the conventional grocery store. The toasted oil just has a more distinctive flavour.

**I have a hard time remembering to drink enough water — do you have any tips or tricks? How do I know if I'm getting enough?** Try leaving a big jug out where you can see it and make sure it's gone by bedtime. Lemon and cucumber slices can help with taste. As long as your urine is pale and you aren't feeling constipated or dehydrated you are probably doing okay (i.e., no headaches, cracked lips, extra dry skin, dry mouth, et cetera).

**I thought I'd be extra "regular" with all these veggies in my diet, but I am actually finding myself a bit constipated. What's up with that?** When you increase your fibre, you also need to increase your water, and if you don't increase it enough, you may end up "plugged up." Here's why: think of soluble fibre as a sponge. If you put that sponge in a pipe (your colon) and pour a little water on top, the sponge will absorb the water, swell up and get stuck in the pipe. How do you get that sponge to move? Pour a bunch more water on top and flush it through! If you are constipated, double your water intake and that will likely make all the difference.

**I need to travel for work and/or entertain clients at restaurants often. How can I manage this and still eat well and lose weight?** Going on the road or out of town for work might make healthy eating more challenging, but with a little planning it's always doable. You'll need to take control over whatever meals and snacks you can, and just do your best with the rest. See Travelling for Work (pages 211–213) for some great tips

| MONDAY | TUESDAY | WEDNESDAY | |
|--------|---------|-----------|---|
| breakfast: | breakfast: | breakfast: | |
| lunch: | lunch: | lunch: | |
| eat at:<br><br>evening activity: | eat at:<br><br>evening activity: | eat at:<br><br>evening activity: | |
| dinner: | dinner: | dinner: | |
| evening prep: | evening prep: | evening prep: | |
| snacks: | snacks: | snacks: | |

# Meal Plan

| THURSDAY | FRIDAY | SATURDAY | SUNDAY |
|----------|--------|----------|--------|
| breakfast: | breakfast: | breakfast: | breakfast: |
| lunch: | lunch: | lunch: | lunch: |
| eat at:<br><br>evening activity: | eat at:<br><br>evening activity: | eat at:<br><br>evening activity: | eat at:<br><br>evening activity: |
| dinner: | dinner: | dinner: | dinner: |
| evening prep: | evening prep: | evening prep: | evening prep: |
| snacks: | snacks: | snacks: | snacks: |

# ACKNOWLEDGEMENTS

Huge thanks to my tasters, big and small, and especially my core group of clients, who encourage me to keep building my program and recipes and who inspire me daily with their personal successes and belief in the power of real food — you know who you are.

For the pinch of love in all my recipes, I draw daily on my own three loving, steadfast and honest taste-testers: Rob, Duncan and Georgia. Thanks for being my biggest cheerleaders and eating what I put in front of you, without wrinkling your noses (much). And thanks for reminding every day of what really matters, so I can keep my own balance in check.

# RECIPE AND INGREDIENT INDEX

# SUBJECT INDEX